T0192744

Register Now for Online Access to Your Book!

SPRINGER PUBLISHING
C**O**NNECT™

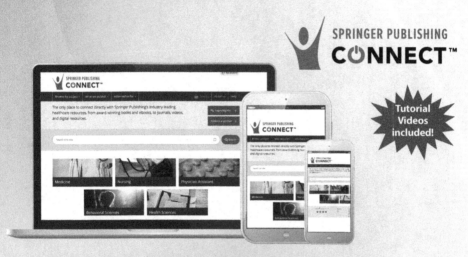

Tutorial Videos included!

Your print purchase of *Improving Financial and Operations Performance* **includes online access to the contents of your book—** increasing accessibility, portability, and searchability!

Access today at:
http://connect.springerpub.com/content/book/978-0-8261-4464-5
or scan the QR code at the right with your smartphone
and enter the access code below.

U0SWEYHB

Scan here for quick access.

If you are experiencing problems accessing the digital component of this product, please contact our customer service department at cs@springerpub.com

The online access with your print purchase is available at the publisher's discretion and may be removed at any time without notice.

Publisher's Note: New and used products purchased from third-party sellers are not guaranteed for quality, authenticity, or access to any included digital components.

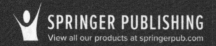

SPRINGER PUBLISHING
View all our products at springerpub.com

"Healthcare is an inherently complex industry. There are many facets that contribute to this, but at healthcare's core, financial performance is often listed as one of the most essential. Of course, patient safety, quality, and efficiency also rise to the top as our industry continues with its transition to value-based care models. However, financial and operational performance are clearly needed before these priority areas are able to deliver optimal outcomes for healthcare delivery. It is on this latter point Dr. Priore's new book focuses and provides such a valuable contribution. Readers will gain deep levels of insight and pragmatic direction for how best to grapple with the complexity of healthcare. As the industry adjusts to its next era, this book is a resource that should not be missed, nor overlooked—make sure to embrace its content with interest and commitment. Facilitating change in healthcare will result."

Peter Angood, MD
President and CEO, American Association for Physician Leadership
Washington, DC

"In today's healthcare environment, it is critical for healthcare leaders to eliminate waste and liberate every possible dollar for direct patient care. Rich Priore gives operations teams and those new to healthcare finance a 'how to' instruction manual from the basics of healthcare finance to developing business cases that are fiscally sound."

Michael Allen, CPA, MHA, FHFMA
Chair, Healthcare Financial Management Association (HFMA)
Chief Financial Offer, OSF Healthcare
Peoria, Illinois

"Dr. Priore's book comes at a critical and challenging time for healthcare organizations and systems, many of which are struggling financially as a result of a pandemic and at the same time facing increasing pressure to demonstrate value for their services. As the past chair of the Association of University Programs in Health Administration (AUPHA) dedicated to improving health and healthcare delivery by developing strong leaders through excellence in healthcare management, this work bridges the common gap between theory and application through real world cases, useful tips, and practical tools. Dr. Priore's long tenure 'in the trenches' enabled him to provide this invaluable resource for planning, assessing, managing, and monitoring optimal financial and operational performance regardless of the size of the organization or the healthcare sector it serves."

Mark L. Diana, PhD
Past Chair, Association of University Programs in
Health Administration (AUPHA)
Professor, Department of Health Policy and Management
School of Public Health and Tropical Medicine
Tulane University
New Orleans, Louisiana

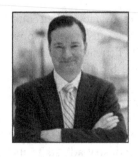

Richard J. Priore, ScD, MHA, FACHE, FACMPE, is a leading international expert on health system transformation. The intersection of his extensive professional and academic backgrounds lends both a relevant industry perspective and an objective evidence-based management approach to driving measurable operational efficiency and expanded capacity for profitable growth and reducing unnecessary waste and cost. Dr. Priore's leadership experience spans more than 27 years in the investor-owned for-profit, private not-for-profit, and government healthcare sectors with senior executive roles in integrated and academic health systems, physician-owned specialty hospitals, and large multispecialty group practices.

Dr. Priore has served as the CEO for several investor-owned hospitals and as a turnaround expert and managing director for the Hunter Group. As a regional executive for a five-hospital health system, he was a principal architect of the Centers for Medicare & Medicaid Services Acute Care Episode Demonstration project that pioneered shared savings and bundled payment policies and programs that incentivize providers to eliminate unnecessary services, improve coordination of care, and achieve better outcomes. Dr. Priore is the Founder, President, and CEO for Excelsior HealthCare Group, an outcomes-driven international management consulting firm specializing in the rapid assessment, focus on execution, and speed of measurable results in improving organizational performance through engaging and aligning the interests of key stakeholders.

Dr. Priore is a Distinguished Service Professor of management, finance, and economics in the Opus College of Business at the University of St. Thomas in St. Paul. He has taught and guest lectured adult learners at more than a dozen accredited universities and colleges. He is a frequent national speaker and facilitator of education and training programs for leading healthcare organizations, Fortune 500 companies, and associations including the Association of American Medical Colleges, American Association of Physician Leadership, American College of Medical Practice Executives, and the American College of Healthcare Executives for which he is faculty and teaches several 2-day seminars, including *Integrating Quality and Cost in a Pay-for-Value Era, Making the Business Case for Quality,* and *Closing the Gap in Physician Engagement, Alignment, and Integration in a Value-Based Environment.*

He earned a doctorate in Health Systems Management from Tulane University, the oldest U.S. school of public health, and a masters in Healthcare Administration from Baylor University. He is board certified in healthcare management and a Fellow in the American College of Healthcare Executives (FACHE) and a Certified Medical Practice Executive and Fellow in the American College of Medical Practice Executives (FACMPE). He is a proud U.S. Army veteran with tours of duty in Europe, Southeast Asia, and Washington, DC, where he served in the White House under two administrations.

Improving Financial and Operations Performance

A Healthcare Leader's Guide

Richard J. Priore, ScD, MHA, FACHE, FACMPE

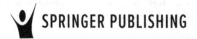

SPRINGER PUBLISHING

Springer Publishing Company, LLC
11 West 42nd Street, New York, NY 10036
www.springerpub.com
connect.springerpub.com/

Acquisitions Editor: David D'Addona
Compositor: Amnet Systems

ISBN: 978-0-8261-4463-8
ebook ISBN: 978-0-8261-4464-5
DOI: 10.1891/9780826144645

Supplemental materials for the chapters and video content for Appendix J are available at **http://connect .springerpub.com/content/book/978-0-8261-4464-5.**

Supplemental material ISBN: 978-0-8261-4465-2

20 21 22 23 24 / 5 4 3 2 1

Library of Congress Cataloging-in-Publication Data
Names: Priore, Richard J., author.
Title: Improving financial and operations performance : a healthcare
  leader's guide / Richard J. Priore.
Description: New York, NY : Springer Publishing Company, [2021] | Includes
  bibliographical references and index. |
Identifiers: LCCN 2020030930 (print) | LCCN 2020030931 (ebook) | ISBN
  9780826144638 (paperback) | ISBN 9780826144645 (ebook)
Subjects: MESH: Health Facility Administration—economics | Financial
  Management—methods | Efficiency, Organizational | Leadership | United
  States
Classification: LCC RA971.3 (print) | LCC RA971.3 (ebook) | NLM WX 157
  AA1 | DDC 362.1068/1—dc23
LC record available at https://lccn.loc.gov/2020030930
LC ebook record available at https://lccn.loc.gov/2020030931

Richard Priore: https://orcid.org/0000-0003-4844-8712

For my beloved mother, Jean. A consummate professional educator whose passion and commitment to learning and teaching never waned throughout her life. Much of this work was written at her hospital bedside deepening my respect and admiration for the front line care team. Indeed health care is a business—a business of taking care of people by highly-skilled and dedicated professionals devoted to helping others.

Contents

PART II PLANNING

3. DEVELOPING THE OPERATING BUDGET   27

PART III ASSESSING

4. CONDUCTING A FINANCIAL CONDITION ANALYSIS: INTERPRETING BASIC FINANCIAL STATEMENTS AND INDICATORS   35

Preface

Healthcare in the United States is undergoing continued and significant turbulence and unprecedented transformation, causing increasing economic and regulatory pressure on provider healthcare organizations' financial and operating performance. The cost of doing business is outstripping flat or decreasing revenue due to traditional inpatient care shifting to an ambulatory setting, reimbursement cuts from both government and commercial payers, and increased operating expenses—impacting the financial well-being of healthcare provider organizations.

In addition to declining reimbursement and softer inpatient volumes, labor and non-labor expenses that account for 80% to 90% of all healthcare provider organizations' costs continue to outpace inflation. The current and projected shortage of nurses and other clinical and technical staff are driving higher labor expense costs as organizations must offer competitive salaries, benefits, and other financial incentives to recruit and retain qualified staff. At the same time, the cost of drugs, supplies, and medical devices continue to increase without commensurate increases in reimbursement. Left unmanaged, these unfavorable trends will force healthcare provider organizations to reduce or eliminate services, impacting quality and access and potentially compromising their ability to provide for the health and wellness needs of the communities they serve.

The market trends threatening healthcare provider organizations require qualified, competent, and confident leaders across all professional backgrounds and all levels of responsibility. Leaders' ability to firmly grasp the financial and operational inner-workings of their healthcare business enterprise and how to effectively manage it supports providing the highest clinical quality, easily accessible, and patient-centered care at the lowest possible cost. Clinical leaders in particular can no longer focus on improving competency in their respective functional expertise without at least a basic understanding of the business of healthcare. Moreover, clinical leaders' financial acumen enables an effective dialogue and productive working relationship with both non-clinical leaders and their peers serving as important boundary spanners.

This book lies at the intersection of leadership effectiveness, performance improvement, operations efficiency, and financial management. It is the product of extensive field work in countless healthcare provider organizations with shared insight from seasoned healthcare leaders. It is based upon five key premises:

1. Leaders are accountable for the financial and operations performance of their organizations.

2. Financial and operations management is a significant challenge to improving organizational performance.

3. Effective financial and operations management skills enable effective leadership and decision-making.

4. Leaders have significant influence over their organizations' financial and operations performance, yet are not effectively trained or given adequate resources.

5. Healthcare is a business—a business of caring for people with growing demands on increasingly scarce resources.

The primary purpose of this book is to provide a practical and applicable approach to understanding and improving financial and operations performance through sharing effective tips, tools, and techniques based on "real world" challenges. Key terms and concepts are presented in easy-to-understand language. Each major topic includes a detailed illustration of a relevant scenario with step-by-step instructions for leaders to apply within their own organization. Toward that critical aim, a common case study organization, Regional Health System (RHS), is used throughout the book with financial and operations data, clear examples, and application of the methods and processes provided that can be translated to any **business enterprise**, the nomenclature used throughout the book referring to any entity over which a leader has financial responsibility and accountability—from a small clinical program, to an outpatient clinic or service, to a large hospital or integrated delivery system.

The book is laid out using a logical and sequential flow of information with major sections that follow the four continuous phases of the Effective Financial and Operations Management Cycle: Planning, Assessing, Managing, and Monitoring. Part I (Introduction) sets the stage for how the current and anticipated future landscape will continue to challenge the performance of healthcare provider organizations and why leaders at all levels need to have a strong understanding and ability to apply a framework for effective financial and operations management. Chapter 1 introduces the transformation to value-based care, the role of leaders in effective financial and operations management, and the challenges they will face. Chapter 2 offers an overview of how money typically flows through the healthcare provider organization and introduces how to measure financial performance or profitability.

Part II (Planning) presents how to develop a basic operating budget, the primary planning tool that provides leaders guidance for monitoring their business enterprise and the overall healthcare provider organization's strategic and financial goals (Chapter 3). Part III (Assessing) begins with Chapter 4 on how to read and interpret common financial statements, financial ratios, and operating indicators to conduct a thorough financial condition analysis. Chapter 5 introduces how to identify and manage financial and operating variances from the goals established during the Planning phase.

Part IV (Managing) provides leaders with proven approaches and examples for improving financial and operations performance, including managing labor productivity and expense (Chapter 6), managing non-labor productivity and expense (Chapter 7), and growing profitable volume and market share (Chapter 8). The final part, Part V (Monitoring), introduces how to make a business case for improving quality (Chapter 9), how to benchmark to improve organizational performance, and how to evaluate the financial impact of a future project (Chapter 10). The end-of-chapter Calls to Action summarize the critical actions required by leaders to drive continuous improvement within their organizations. Electronic templates are provided as an additional resource for leaders to support ease of application. Supplemental materials for the chapters and video content for Appendix J are available at connect.springerpub.com/content/book/978-0-8261-4464-5.

This book was written for both new and experienced healthcare leaders who want a leg-up to better understand and successfully tackle the myriad of complex challenges within their organizations. Admittedly, the first part is relatively basic and intended for newer leaders to level-set their understanding of health care and financial management. The later parts are more advanced and complex in scope. While the book is designed using a building block approach, each chapter can be used as a standalone lesson.

Richard J. Priore

PART I

INTRODUCTION

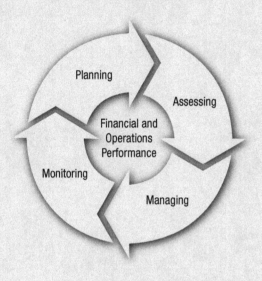

CHAPTER 1

INTRODUCTION TO EFFECTIVE HEALTHCARE FINANCIAL AND OPERATIONS MANAGEMENT

LEARNING OBJECTIVES

- Explain the key drivers impacting the financial and operations performance of healthcare provider organizations.
- Define the role of healthcare leaders in the effective financial and operations management of healthcare provider organizations.
- List the challenges to effective financial and operations management.

KEY TERMS AND CONCEPTS

Value-based care

Fee-for-service

Capitation

Bundled payment

Pay-for-performance (P4P)

Shared savings

Value

Lagging indicator

Leading indicator

INTRODUCTION

The current healthcare operating environment is causing leaders responsible for the financial well-being of their organizations to think and act differently. National healthcare costs continue to rise, consuming nearly 20% of the gross domestic product. Among the many contributors to the unsustainable escalating cost trend are overtreatment, missed prevention opportunities, unwarranted clinical variation, and a lack of coordination of care largely stemming from the current payment system that rewards the quantity of services delivered rather than quality.[1] As the healthcare industry makes the transition from paying for volume to paying for value healthcare leaders must understand the business of healthcare to successfully navigate their organizations through these uncertain and austere times.

MOVEMENT TO VALUE-BASED CARE

According to the American Hospital Association, the healthcare industry will ultimately shift from the "first curve" where healthcare provider organizations operate largely in a volume-based, acute care focused, and fee-for-service environment with little financial risk to the "second curve" where they will be building **value-based care** systems and business models marked by realigned payment incentives for quality and efficiency, population health management, and shared risk. Most healthcare provider organizations are presently in a transition period known as "life in the gap" between the first and second curves.[2] The primary catalyst for the value-based movement was the federal government through the Centers for Medicare & Medicaid Services' (CMS) goal to reduce unwarranted clinical variation, waste, and unnecessary expense from the predominant payment-for-volume reimbursement model. The CMS announced its goal to have 90% of Medicare payments tied to quality outcomes and 50% tied to alternative payment models, such as accountable care organizations and bundled payments, by 2018—an ambitious and unrecognized goal.[3] Regardless of the origin or current drivers, the evolving value-based math for how healthcare provider organizations get paid means they must learn to do much more with significantly less.

IMPACT OF REIMBURSEMENT MODELS ON UTILIZATION OF SERVICES AND PAYMENT

Despite the movement toward value-based care, most of the money currently paid to healthcare provider organizations is tied to volume. How healthcare provider organizations are reimbursed drives their incentives and profitability. The **fee-for-service** or case rate reimbursement model promotes a "churn and earn" mentality where providers are financially rewarded for doing more, even if unnecessary and non-value added. Alternatively, **capitation** provides a fixed amount for providing services, typically for a large population or employer group, a specified set of services, or for an entire episode of care like a **bundled payment** for total joint replacements.

Capitation often includes quality improvement goals where the financial incentive for the healthcare provider organization is to limit or reduce unnecessary or wasteful care. Moving toward the "second curve," including population health management, will require healthcare provider organizations' sharing some financial risk through some form of **pay-for-performance** or **shared savings** for achieving specified quality performance improvement goals that reduce waste and unnecessary cost. The various common reimbursement models and their influence on healthcare provider organization financial incentives are provided in Table 1.1.

THE ROLE OF HEALTHCARE LEADERS IN EFFECTIVE FINANCIAL AND OPERATIONS MANAGEMENT

The traditional role of healthcare leaders in the effective financial and operations management of the healthcare provider organization is to plan for, acquire, and use resources to maximize clinical effectiveness and operational efficiency. This cycle requires leaders to be accountable for continuously monitoring and improving financial and operations performance. Leaders must gain insight from the available financial and operational data to make informed decisions that support the organization's strategy and goals (Figure 1.1). Beyond the traditional role, healthcare leaders must define, measure, and continuously improve **value** in their organization, where value equals quality divided by cost—two variables that are inextricably linked (Box 1.1).

What's more, leaders' basic knowledge and acumen of the financial and operations inner-workings of their healthcare provider organization supports providing high quality, easily accessible, and patient-centered care at the lowest

TABLE 1.1 **Impact of Reimbursement Models**

REIMBURSEMENT MODEL	DEFINITION	FINANCIAL INCENTIVE
Fee-for-Service	Paid fixed fee for every covered service performed	Increase utilization and revenue
Capitation	Set amount paid per person in a specific geographic area or demographic for a pre-determined set of services	Limit utilization and expenses
Bundled Payments	Negotiated fixed payments for specific episodes of care	Limit or decrease utilization and expenses
Pay-for-Performance	Paid bonus to achieve specified performance measure targets	Achieve compliance to measures
Shared Savings	Share a percent of cost savings assuming no decrement to quality	Limit or decrease utilization and expenses

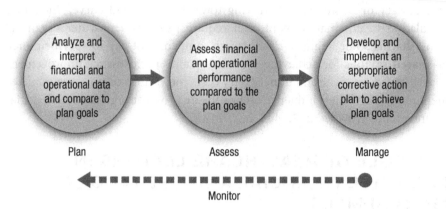

FIGURE 1.1 Role of healthcare leaders in effective financial management.

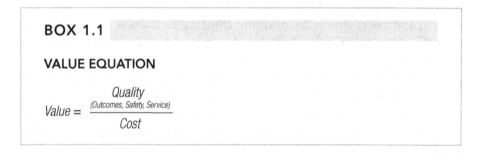

BOX 1.1

VALUE EQUATION

$$Value = \frac{Quality_{\ (Outcomes,\ Safety,\ Service)}}{Cost}$$

possible cost. Quality performance improvement measures are the leading indicators and the resulting financial impact is the lagging indicator. Regardless of an organization's ownership or tax status, it must maintain a positive bottom line to sustain its mission. According to the late Sister Irene Kraus, "No margin, no mission."[4] Healthcare leaders' financial acumen also enables an effective dialogue and productive working relationship among clinical and administrative leaders.

CHALLENGES TO EFFECTIVE FINANCIAL AND OPERATIONS MANAGEMENT

Effective financial and operations management is both an art and a science in any industry; however, it is particularly so in healthcare due to the inherent challenges created by three conditions. First, there is dynamic change and uncertainty with evolving payment models. Second, there is a dearth of accurate and actionable data. Third, leaders are not adequately prepared or given the appropriate resources to understand and interpret financial data in order to make timely and informed decisions.

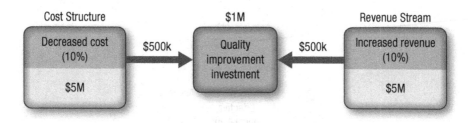

FIGURE 1.2 Link between quality improvement and financial performance.

Financial and operations management is like driving a car with foggy windows—making imperfect decisions with imperfect information, and just as risky. The imperative for healthcare leaders' effective financial and operations management transcends improving organizational profitability. Gone are the days where administrative and clinical leaders have separate roles and responsibilities based on their respective expertise. Today all healthcare leaders must understand and apply the tools of effective financial and operations management to improve organizational performance to support their mission and achieve their strategic goals.

In the simple illustration provided in Figure 1.2, assume the leader can reduce unnecessary expense by 10%, such as through streamlining processes that eliminate waste, without compromising quality. The additional capacity created from increasing efficiency enables the ability to increase volume and market share adding another 10% in new revenue. The resulting financial impact (**lagging indicator**) and by-product from the effort creates $1 million that can be invested to further achieving the organization's quality performance improvement goals (**leading indicator**).

PHASES OF EFFECTIVE FINANCIAL AND OPERATIONS MANAGEMENT

The four continuous Phases of Effective Financial and Operations Management are Planning, Assessing, Managing, and Monitoring, as shown in Figure 1.3.

Planning

The first phase of Effective Financial and Operations Management is Planning. Planning is the formal process to identify and prioritize the organization's goals to support its mission. Short-range goals are typically less than 1 year. Mid-range goals are usually 1 to 3 years and long-range are more than 3 years. Budgeting (Chapter 3) is the most important process to identify and prioritize the financial resources required to achieve the organization's goals.

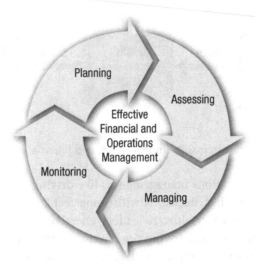

FIGURE 1.3 Phases of effective financial and operations management.

Assessing

Assessing is the continuous process to compare the goals identified in Planning with the actual performance of the organization by conducting a financial condition analysis (Chapter 4) that includes reviewing and interpreting financial statements, financial ratios, and operating indicators.

Managing

Managing includes the range of actions taken by healthcare leaders to guide and drive measurable change to achieve the performance improvement opportunities identified during Assessing. Effectively managing financial and operations performance involves understanding the specific drivers of performance and then developing and decisively implementing a plan to achieve the organization's goals.

Monitoring

Finally, continuously Monitoring the results from the actions taken in Managing and then comparing them to internal and external benchmarks, such as a balanced scorecard or performance measurement dashboard, enables leaders to anticipate required actions rather than react to unexpected changes.

SUMMARY

The anticipated healthcare landscape will continue to challenge and pressure healthcare provider organizations' bottom line, impacting the ability to sustain their mission. The transformation to value-based care will require demonstrating high quality outcomes and superior patient experience while reducing waste and unnecessary expense. To navigate the uncertain and austere future, healthcare leaders must drive quality performance improvement and strong financial performance through effective financial and operations management.

CALLS TO ACTION

Leaders should:

- Understand the changing reimbursement models and their impact on financial and operations performance.
- Improve their financial and operations management acumen to achieve their organization's mission
- Apply a deliberate framework for planning, assessing, managing, and monitoring financial and operations performance.

References

1. Porter ME, Kaplan RS. How to pay for health care. *Harvard Business Review*. 2016;94(7-8):88-98, 100, 134.
2. American Hospital Association, Committee on Research. *Your Hospital's Path to the Second Curve: Integration and Transformation*. Health Research & Educational Trust; 2014.
3. Centers for Medicare and Medicaid. Better Care. Smarter Spending. Healthier People: Paying Providers for Value, Not Volume. CMS.gov Newsroom. January 26, 2015 https://www.cms.gov/newsroom/fact-sheets/better-care-smarter-spending-healthier-people-paying-providers-value-not-volume.
4. Langley M. Money order: Nuns' zeal for profits shapes hospital chain, wins fans. *Wall Street Journal*. January 7, 1998.

CHAPTER 2

HOW MONEY FLOWS THROUGH A HEALTHCARE PROVIDER ORGANIZATION

LEARNING OBJECTIVES

- Describe common key terms and concepts used in financial management.
- Explain how money typically flows through a healthcare provider organization.
- Apply common measures to assess the high-level financial performance of a business enterprise.
- Calculate the breakeven point.

TOOLS AND TECHNIQUES

- Profitability analysis
- Breakeven analysis

KEY TERMS AND CONCEPTS

Revenue cycle

Gross charges

Payer

Charge data master (CDM)

Net revenue

Contractual adjustment

Patient obligation

Cost shifting

Fixed expense

Variable expense

Direct expense

Indirect expense

Overhead expense

Net income

Profitability analysis

Loss

Profit

Operating margin

Earnings before interest, taxes, depreciation, and amortization (EBITDA)

Breakeven

INTRODUCTION

Effective financial management requires leaders' having a basic knowledge and ability to comfortably use the "language of finance." The key terms and concepts listed in this chapter, at a minimum, should be adopted into leaders' vocabularies, with the understanding that there are different terms that can be used to mean the same thing and are often used interchangeably. The best way to introduce these key terms and concepts is to walk through how money typically flows through a healthcare provider organization, sometimes referred to as the **revenue cycle**. Later in the chapter, two important techniques will be presented for conducting a high-level profitability analysis to determine the financial performance or well-being of a business enterprise with application through the Regional Health System case.

HOW MONEY FLOWS THROUGH A HEALTHCARE PROVIDER ORGANIZATION

The illustration presented in Figure 2.1 shows the basic four-step process that occurs after the healthcare provider organization delivers a service to a patient that includes sending the bill to the payer, collecting payment, paying expenses, and determining profitability.

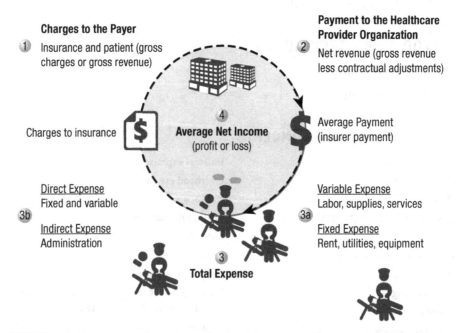

FIGURE 2.1 How money flows through a healthcare provider organization.

① Charges to the Payer

Gross charges or gross revenue is the amount that the healthcare provider organization bills the payer for patient care and related services. A **payer** (or payor) is the entity, such as Medicare or private insurance, or the individual responsible for paying the bill. There can be multiple payers for every bill, such as if the patient has Medicare and additional private insurance, plus the amount the patient is obligated to pay. Payers include the government, such as Medicare and Medicaid, or commercial health insurers, such as United Healthcare, Aetna, and Humana. Employers are also payers through the portion of employee healthcare costs they cover. Individual employees are also payers through their contribution to the final bill in the form of premiums deducted from their paycheck, co-pays, and deductibles. Taxpayers ultimately foot the bill for healthcare services through the portion of their wages allocated for government entitlement programs and in lieu of higher wages from their employer.

Healthcare provider organizations are required to use a single and standard fee schedule or fixed pricing for their services, similar to a menu at a restaurant. The fee schedule is known as the **charge data master** (CDM). Healthcare provider organizations can only have one price list for their services. Therefore, they typically charge much more than what they expect to eventually receive, knowing that the payment will be whittled down as members with insurance receive a discount from the total bill. Typically, patients without any insurance are charged and expected to pay the full amount; however, organizations will often negotiate a discount for prompt payment or allow the patient to pay their bill in installments over a period of time.

② Payment to the Healthcare Provider Organization

The amount of the total fee that the healthcare provider organization actually collects from the payer is **net revenue**, also net operating revenue. This is the actual amount or reimbursement that the organization receives. Similar to the sticker price on a new car at a dealer, most payers do not pay the full price or the total billed charges. The final amount paid is based on the negotiation and formal contract between the healthcare provider organization and the commercial payers. The difference between the billed and the negotiated amounts is the **contractual adjustment**, also called a discount or write off.

The total amount received by the healthcare provider organization varies and is determined by several factors including the qualification of the charge (or claim), the type of insurance coverage the patient has, and the amount collected that is owed by the patient after the final insurance payment has been processed, known as the **patient obligation**. This is often referred to as the

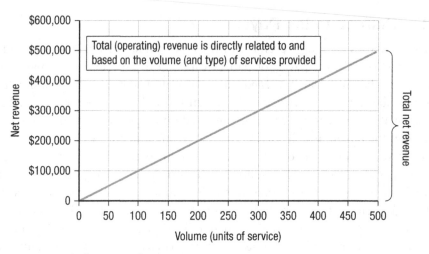

FIGURE 2.2 Calculating total net revenue.

patient responsibility or burden. The total operating revenue is directly related to, and based on, the volume and type of services provided shown in Figure 2.2.

On average, governmental payers reimburse less than what the services cost the healthcare provider organization, as shown in Figure 2.3. This is due to the combination of healthcare provider organization's higher than necessary operating expenses from waste and inefficiency and from shrinking reimbursement from federal and state reform efforts to reduce healthcare expenditures. Because organizations deliver services to these payers at a loss, they expect to make up the difference on the higher-reimbursing commercial payers, known as **cost shifting**. However, in recent years commercial payer organizations have been limiting cost shifting efforts.

③ Expense

Fixed and Variable Expense

Operating expense includes four categories: labor, supplies, purchased services, and other. The typical allocation of total operating expense is shown in Figure 2.4. At least three quarters or more of the total operating expense for a healthcare provider organization is from labor and non-labor expense (staff and stuff). Labor expense includes the salary, wages, and benefits paid to employees. Non-labor expense includes the supplies used to provide services, such as medical supplies, drugs, and implantable devices. Purchased services includes the range of the services needed for delivering care, such as contracts with anesthesiology and other providers, biomedical equipment maintenance, and consulting. Other expenses include insurance, depreciation, research, and teaching.

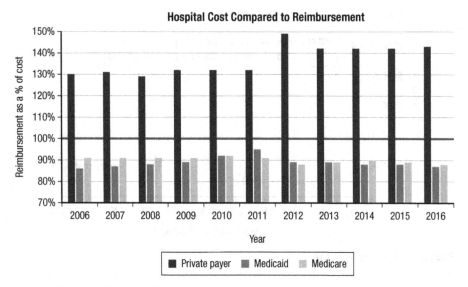

Hospital Cost Compared to Reimbursement

FIGURE 2.3 Healthcare provider organization cost versus reimbursement for government and commercial payers.

SOURCE: Data from the American Hospital Association. *Trendwatch Chartbook 2019: Trends in Hospital Financing. Aggregate Hospital Payment-to-Cost Ratios for Private Payers, Medicare, and Medicaid, 1995-2016.* American Hospital Association; 2019.

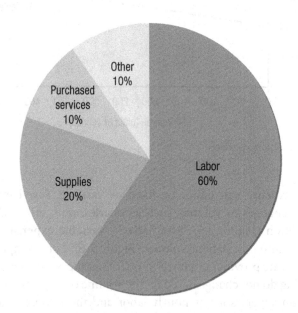

FIGURE 2.4 Where money is spent in healthcare provider organizations.

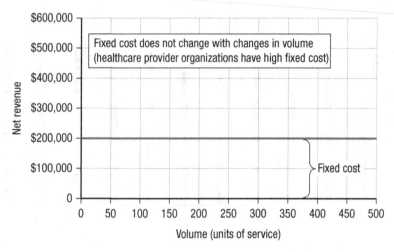

FIGURE 2.5 Fixed expense.

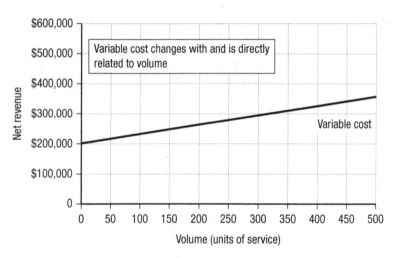

FIGURE 2.6 Variable expense.

Operating expense can either be fixed or variable. **Fixed expense** does not vary with changes in volume, such as salaries, rent, utilities, and equipment depreciation (Figure 2.5). Alternatively, **variable expense** increases or decreases depending on patient volume (Figure 2.6). For example, the salary paid to a healthcare provider organization's CEO or the annual amount paid for groundskeeping do not change based on the volume of patients seen. However, the cost of non-supervisory or hourly labor and most supplies and services have a direct relationship with and vary according to the number of patients seen.

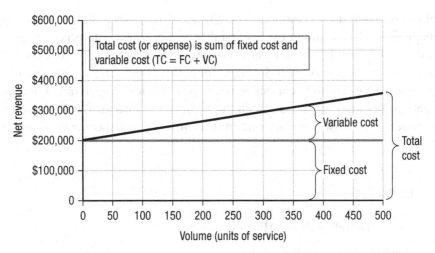

FIGURE 2.7 Total expense.

The total operating expense or total cost (TC) is calculated by fixed cost (FC) and variable cost (VC) as shown in Figure 2.7.

Direct, Indirect, and Overhead Expense

In addition to expenses being either fixed or variable, they can also be classified as direct, indirect, or overhead. **Direct expense** is tied to providing services, such as nursing care, expendable medical supplies, drugs, and food. **Indirect expense** is for providing patient care support and services that typically do not involve "hands on" care, such as the clinical laboratory, biomedical engineering, facility maintenance, and housekeeping. **Overhead expense**, sometimes referred to as "fully loaded" expense, is typically fixed and includes the cost for management support and services to run the organization, including executive salaries, human resources, marketing, and legal fees.

④ Net Income

The remaining amount after all expenses have been covered is **net income**. Net income can be expressed as a percentage, known as the operating margin, which will be covered later.

CONDUCTING A PROFITABILITY ANALYSIS

Profitability is the most important component of any business. According to economist Milton Friedman, "There is one and only one social responsibility of business—to use its resources and engage in activities designed to increase its profit…"[1] Determining the profitability of a business enterprise, program, service, or provider is a critical action to enable leaders' clear understanding if the entity is making or losing money. This allows further assessment to determine the need for a corrective action plan. Conducting an initial or quick **profitability analysis** or assessment of the business enterprise is calculated by subtracting expense from revenue to determine the net income, as shown in Box 2.1.

BOX 2.1

CALCULATING PROFITABILITY

Revenue − Expense = Net income

Net income can also be expressed as a ratio of the amount of operating expense required to generate operating revenue. The formula for this ratio, known as **operating margin**, shown in Box 2.2, is operating revenues less operating costs divided by operating revenue. The resulting calculation is then multiplied by 100, because operating margin is always expressed as a percentage. Operating margin will be discussed further in Chapter 4. For-profit organizations often use a different calculation for profitability, known as **earnings before interest, taxes, depreciation, and amortization** or EBITDA.

BOX 2.2

CALCULATING OPERATING MARGIN FORMULA

$$\text{Operating margin} = \frac{\text{Operating revenue} - \text{Operating expense}}{\text{Operating revenue}} \times 100$$

The relationship between revenue and expense is shown in Figure 2.8. Total net revenue, the money collected by the organization, is represented by the upward sloping light gray line ① expressing the direct (positive) relationship between volume and revenue. Typically, the more volume of complex services that an organization provides, such as inpatient admissions, diagnostic tests, clinic visits, and surgeries, the more money it makes. Total expense or cost is represented by both the dark gray horizontal line ② for the fixed expense and

TABLE 2.1 **Different Ways to Show Negative Financial Numbers**

INDICATOR	DESCRIPTION
−$000	Negative sign
($000)	Parentheses
$000	Red number

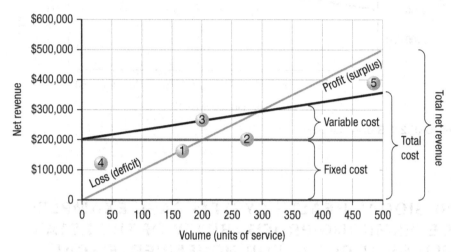

FIGURE 2.8 Relationship between revenue and expense to determine profitability.

the black upward sloping line ③ for the variable expense. When total operating expense exceeds total revenue it is a **loss** or deficit ④, while total expense less than the total net revenue collected results in a **profit** or surplus ⑤.

In financial management terms, a negative amount can be expressed several different ways; including a negative sign, in red, or within parentheses as shown in Table 2.1.

BREAKEVEN ANALYSIS

Another quick measure of profitability is **breakeven** (or breakeven point), particularly to assess the financial viability of a specific project or initiative. The breakeven point is where the total net revenue minus the total operating expense equals zero, as shown in Figure 2.9 ⑥. Determining the breakeven point is useful to understand the minimum amount of volume required where the project or service will not lose any money in the short run. In the long run, factoring inflation and the time value of money, covered in Chapter 10, could cause the project, service, or organization to lose money.

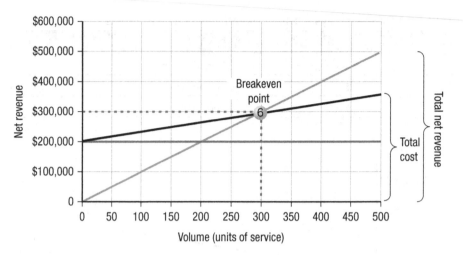

FIGURE 2.9 Breakeven point.

REGIONAL HEALTH SYSTEM CASE EXAMPLE: DETERMINING PROFITABILITY OF THE RETAIL FLU SHOT CLINIC FOR NOVEMBER, FISCAL YEAR 20X2

To lend context to the key terms and concepts presented it will be instructive to walk through a practical example of how money flows through a healthcare provider organization to calculate profitability using information and data provided on Regional Health System's (RHS) retail flu shot clinic. RHS has a contracted rate with Medicare, Medicaid, and most major commercial insurance companies to provide flu shots. In November, the clinic administered shots to 400 adults and 700 children. The clinic charges $50 per flu shot (gross charge), according to its published fee schedule. The average payment (net revenue) it receives from all of its payers combined is $20. Otherwise, patients without insurance must pay the full charge.

The variable expense for RHS to provide flu shots includes a licensed practical nurse, who administers the shot, and the supplies. The cost of the nurse is $7.20 per shot based on the total labor expense divided by the annual volume of shots administered. The cost of supplies per shot is $6.50 and includes the flu vaccine, syringe, alcohol prep, 2 × 2 gauze, and bandage. The fixed cost to provide the shot is $4.50 and includes rent for the clinic space and utilities, such as electricity and water. Clinic operating costs are summarized in Table 2.2.

TABLE 2.2 **Regional Health System's Flu Shot Clinic Operating Expense**

OPERATING EXPENSE	TYPE	COST PER SHOT
Nursing	Variable	$7.20
Supplies	Variable	$6.50
Rent and utilities	Fixed	$4.50
	Total Cost per Shot	$18.20

What Is the Profitability of the Flu Shot Clinic in November? Did It Make or Lose Money?

Applying the basic formula:

$$\text{Revenue} - \text{Expense} = \text{Net income}$$

Where revenue:

$$400 \text{ adults} + 700 \text{ children} = 1{,}100 \text{ total shots administered}$$
$$1{,}100 \text{ shots} \times \$20 \text{ average net revenue} = \$22{,}000$$

And expense:

$$1{,}100 \text{ shots} \times \$18.20 \text{ total cost per shot} = \$20{,}020$$

Net income can then be calculated:

$$\$22{,}000 \text{ (Revenue)} - \$20{,}020 \text{ (Expense)} = \$1{,}980 \text{ (Net Income)}$$

The net income, or money that's left after paying expenses, was positive. Therefore the clinic was profitable in November. How profitable the clinic was compared to other business enterprises can be determined using the calculation for operating margin:

$$\text{Operating margin} = \frac{\text{Operating revenue} - \text{Operating expense}}{\text{Operating revenue}} \times 100$$

$$\text{Operating margin} = \frac{\$22{,}000 - \$20{,}020}{\$22{,}000} \times 100$$

$$= \frac{\$1{,}980}{\$22{,}000} \times 100 \text{ (note that the numerator is the net income)}$$

$$= 9.0\% \text{ For every \$1 spent on expense, it made \$.09 in profit.}$$

Using the figure previously presented on how money flows through the healthcare provider organization, let's walk through the basic profitability

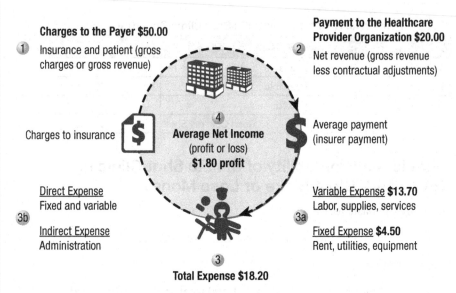

FIGURE 2.10 How money flows through the RHS flu shot clinic.

calculations for an individual patient (Figure 2.10). The gross charge to the payer ($50) minus the contractual allowance or discount ($30) is the payment or net revenue received ($20). Subtracting total expenses ($18.20) from the total revenue ($20) is the net income ($1.80) per patient. Recall that net income can also be expressed as a percentage, known as the operating margin (9%). The source data for this Case Example is available on Springer Connect (visit connect .springerpub.com/content/book/978-0-8261-4464-5/chapter/ch02 and access the show chapter supplementary dropdown at the beginning of the chapter).

SUMMARY

Healthcare leaders must understand and speak the "language of finance" to enable productive conversations to support achieving their organizations' financial goals. Knowing and applying the business of healthcare terms, such as revenue, expense, and net income are essential for effective financial management. Leaders can apply common profitability measure calculations to continuously assess the financial well-being of their business enterprise.

CALLS TO ACTION

Leaders should:

- Adopt the "language of finance."

- Apply the basic calculations for profitability (net income, operating margin, and breakeven point).
- Continuously assess the profitability of their business enterprise.

Reference

1. Friedman M. The social responsibility of business is to increase its profits. *The New York Times Magazine*. September 13, 1970.

PART II

PLANNING

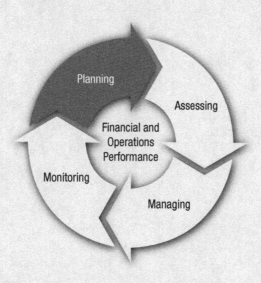

INTRODUCTION TO PLANNING

The first phase of Effective Financial and Operations Management is Planning. Planning is the formal process to identify and prioritize the organization's goals to support its mission. Short-range goals are typically less than 1 year. Mid-range goals are usually 1 to 3 years and long-range are more than 3 years. The operating budget is the most important tool used to identify and prioritize the financial resources required to support the organization's mission and achieve its strategic goals.

CHAPTER 3

DEVELOPING THE OPERATING BUDGET

LEARNING OBJECTIVES

- Describe the different types of budgets and their purpose.
- Recall a typical budgeting process.
- Apply the process to develop the operating budget.

TOOLS AND TECHNIQUES

- Operating budget

KEY TERMS AND CONCEPTS

Fiscal year (FY)	Revenue budget
Budget	Expense budget
Operating budget	Cash budget
Statistical budget	Capital budget

INTRODUCTION

Similar and complementary to strategic planning, financial planning supports the organization's mission and goals by forecasting revenue and expenses over a specified period of time, typically a fiscal year. A **fiscal year** (FY) is used for accounting purposes to define when the organization's financial activity is measured, which may coincide with the calendar year beginning January 1 and ending December 31. However, not all organizations use the calendar year for their fiscal year. For example, the federal government's fiscal year begins October 1 and ends September 30. The **budget** is a planning tool that provides leaders with guidance for monitoring a business enterprise. Effective budgeting serves four primary purposes:

1. Planning
2. Allocating
3. Communicating
4. Managing

Budgeting is the formal planning process to support the organization's mission and strategic goals and to make sure it can meet its financial obligations. The budget defines how the organization will allocate resources to achieve near-term objectives, such as increasing the number of ambulatory clinics or hiring additional providers to meet expanding patient needs. The final budget is the financial guidance to communicate operational expectations and targets, such as new volume growth. Finally, the budget is the baseline document from which future performance is compared through variance analysis, addressed in Chapter 5.

TYPES OF BUDGETS AND KEY USES

There are several types of budgets used for planning, allocating, communicating, and managing the healthcare provider organization's resources. The common types of budgets, their measurement indicators, and the key activities or actions that influence their development are presented in Table 3.1.

TABLE 3.1 **Types of Budgets**

TYPE	MEASUREMENT INDICATORS	KEY DRIVERS
Statistical budget	Number of discharges, patient days, clinic visits, ancillary tests, surgeries	Market trends, providers, new programs and services, competition
Expense budget	Labor, supplies, purchased services, bad debt	Inflation, vendor agreements, new programs and services, efficiency
Revenue budget	Net revenue (operating, non-operating), contractual allowances	Volume, payer mix and contracts, service mix, coding and documentation
Cash budget	Days cash on-hand, days in accounts receivable, accounts payable	Cash collection policies
Operating budget	Operating income, operating margin	Strategic goals, volume and revenue growth plans, operating efficiency
Capital budget	Interest rates (debt), depreciation	Capital needs (expansion)

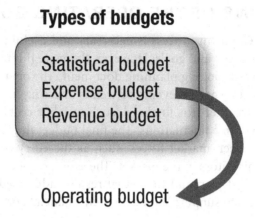

FIGURE 3.1 Developing the operating budget.

The primary and most important budget used by leaders is the operating budget. The **operating budget** is simply a forecast of future revenue and expenses for a specific business enterprise over a specified period of time, such as a year. The operating budget is created from three other separate budgets, shown in Figure 3.1. The **statistical budget** is used to identify all of the various units of service or patient volume statistics—measures that will be used to drive the rest of the budgeting process; for example, historical outpatient clinic volume could be used to estimate the projected number of visits in the coming budget year. Projected reimbursement and payer mix data are used to create the **revenue budget**. Forecasted operating costs are used to develop the **expense budget**. The **cash budget** projects inflow and outflow of money.

BUDGETING PROCESS

Effective budgeting is both an art and a science. Budgeting involves extensive, often complicated, analytical processes that require several levels of review, input, and approval. A typical process to develop the operating budget and the estimated timeline includes several steps.

First, senior leaders provide planning guidance with high-level goals, assumptions, and constraints, usually at least 4 to 6 months before the new fiscal year begins. Then mid-level managers aided by financial staff produce department budgets at least 3 to 4 months before the new fiscal year. Then the individual budgets are aggregated, negotiated, and reconciled with organizational goals at least 2 to 3 months before the new fiscal year begins. The final budget is then presented to the board or governing authority for final approval before publication to all organizational leaders.

LIMITATIONS OF THE OPERATING BUDGET

The budget development process is necessary and useful for supporting the organization's strategy and goals. However, there are limitations because the budget is a forward-looking planning document. The operating budget does not account for unexpected events or trends affecting financial and operations performance after it is finalized, such as labor costs increases, supply shortages, and volume fluctuations. The final budget may not take into consideration unforeseen market forces, such as the entry or exit of referring providers or competitors in the market. Therefore, reconciling the difference between the budget plan and the actual results, addressed in Chapter 5, is critical for leaders to support achieving their financial goals.

CAPITAL BUDGET

Another common type of budget that leaders may encounter and be asked to develop or contribute to is the capital budget. As the name implies, the **capital budget** is developed for high-dollar items, such as new equipment and facilities. The capital budget development process is similar to the operating budget and supports more long-term strategic goals. Big-ticket item projects or initiatives, such as purchasing a new or replacing an outdated CT scanner, should involve forecasting the financial impact over a period of time, typically 3 to 5 years. The critical process for identifying the financial impact of a future project is addressed in Chapter 10.

REGIONAL HEALTH SYSTEM CASE EXAMPLE: CREATING THE RETAIL FLU SHOT CLINIC'S OPERATING BUDGET

Regional Health System is planning for next year's revenue and expense goals during the annual budgeting process. As part of the process, leadership needs to forecast volume for the retail Flu Shot Clinic. Due to a public health department advertising campaign to increase vaccination rates, the anticipated number of adults and children getting a flu shot is expected to increase by 15%. Also, operating expenses are expected to increase 8% due to an anticipated shortage of the flu vaccine combined with rising labor and supply costs. The CFO has issued budget guidance to all retail clinics to plan for a 10% operating margin. The annual operating budget for FY 20X3 can be prepared using the planning guidance reflected in the statistical budget in Table 3.2 and the expense budget in Table 3.3.

TABLE 3.2 Regional Health System's Flu Shot Clinic Statistical Budget

PATIENT TYPE	HISTORICAL VOLUME FY20X1	PROJECTED VOLUME FY20X2
Adult	400	460
Child	700	805
Total volume	1,100	1,265

TABLE 3.3 Regional Health System's Flu Shot Clinic Expense Budget

OPERATING EXPENSE	FY 20X1		FY 20X2	
	EXPENSE	TOTAL EXPENSE	EXPENSE	TOTAL EXPENSE
Labor				
Salaries	$6,336.00	$7,920.00	$7,286.40	$8,997.12
Benefits (20%)	$1,584.00		$1,710.72	
Supplies				
Flu vaccine	$4,950.00	$7,150.00	$5,544.00	$8,008.00
Medical supplies	$2,200.00		$2,464.00	
Rent and Utilities				
Clinic lease	$4,400.00	$4,950.00	$4,928.00	$5,544.00
Utilities	$550.00		$616.00	
Total Annual Expense		$20,020.00		$22,549.12

Given the projected FY 20X2 volume and expense for the Flu Shot Clinic, the next step is to create the revenue budget, shown in Table 3.4, assuming the contracted reimbursement rate is the same as FY 20X1.

TABLE 3.4 Regional Health System's Flu Shot Clinic Revenue Budget

	FY 20X1	FY20X2
Revenue per shot	$20.00	
Patient volume	1,100	1,265
Total revenue	$22,000.00	$25,300.00

With the completed statistical, expense, and revenue budgets the preliminary operating budget, shown in Table 3.5, can be developed.

Given the projected net income from the preliminary operating budget and recalling the information presented in Chapter 2, does the retail Flu Shot Clinic achieve the CFO's guidance of a 10% operating margin?

To determine if the annual budget guidance is achieved in the proposed budget plan, recall the formula for calculating the operating margin, where:

$$\text{Operating margin} = \frac{\$25{,}300 - \$22{,}549.12}{\$25{,}300} \times 100 = 10.9\%$$

The projected operating margin of 10.9% achieves the budgeted target of 10%.

TABLE 3.5 **Regional Health System's Flu Shot Clinic Operating Budget (Preliminary)**

	FY20X2
Volume	1,265
GROSS REVENUE	$63,250.00
Contractual Discount	($37,950)
NET REVENUE	$25,300.00
EXPENSE	
Labor	$8,997.12
Supplies	$8,008.00
Rent and utilities	$5,544.00
TOTAL EXPENSE	$22,549.12
NET INCOME	$2,750.88

SUMMARY

The first phase of the effective financial and operations management process is Planning. The primary technique for financial planning is budgeting. The operating budget is used to plan, allocate, communicate, and manage organizational resources. Developing the operating budget is a dynamic process. Being able to incorporate new information that affects budget projections is important to develop as reasonably accurate a budget as possible.

CALLS TO ACTION

Leaders should:

- Get involved early and understand their organization's budgeting process.
- Attempt to accurately identify and project volume, expense, and revenue in developing the operating budget.

PART III

ASSESSING

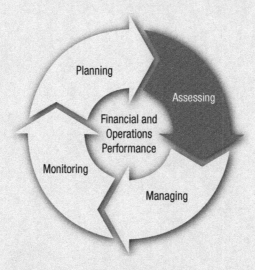

INTRODUCTION TO ASSESSING

Assessing is the continuous process to compare the goals identified in Planning with the actual performance of the business enterprise. The most effective approach to assess performance is conducting a financial condition analysis. The financial condition analysis involves reviewing and making sense of financial statements, operating indicators, and financial ratios to identify and implement opportunities for improvement.

CHAPTER 4

CONDUCTING A FINANCIAL CONDITION ANALYSIS: INTERPRETING BASIC FINANCIAL STATEMENTS AND INDICATORS

LEARNING OBJECTIVES

- Summarize the purpose of basic financial statements.
- Calculate various financial ratios and operating indicators.
- Apply how to interpret data from financial statements, financial ratios, and operating indicators to conduct a financial condition analysis.

TOOLS AND TECHNIQUES

- Financial statement analysis
- Financial ratio analysis
- Operating indicator analysis
- Financial condition analysis

KEY TERMS AND CONCEPTS

Balance sheet	Net assets
Basic accounting equation	Financial ratio analysis
Current assets	Statement of cash flows
Fixed assets	Income statement
Investments	Operating statement
Liabilities	Trend analysis

Comparative analysis

Total margin

Operating margin

Contribution margin

Liquidity ratio

Days cash on hand

Asset management ratios

Total asset turnover ratio

Inventory turnover ratio

Profitability ratios

Price indicators

Volume indicators

Length of stay (LOS) indicators

Intensity of service indicators

Case mix index (CMI)

Medicare severity-diagnosis related group (MS-DRG)

Case mix-adjusted (CMA)

Efficiency indicators

Full-time equivalents (FTE)

Input cost indicators

INTRODUCTION

Conducting a financial condition analysis enables leaders to have a clear understanding of the financial health of their business enterprise. It also provides leaders with actionable information and insight to make timely and effective decisions to achieve the goals of the larger healthcare provider organization. A thorough financial condition analysis assesses whether the organization has the financial capacity and resources to support its mission and achieve its strategic goals. The results of the analysis typically focus on the business's opportunities for improvement relative to the targets set during the budgeting process covered in Chapter 3. Among the common techniques used to conduct the financial condition include the financial statement analysis, financial ratio analysis, and operating indicator analysis.

UNDERSTANDING FINANCIAL STATEMENTS

The first step in the financial condition analysis is to review the available financial statements. Understanding and interpreting basic financial statements allows leaders to identify and prioritize the necessary actions to close any gaps from the budget. Among the most common financial statements, often collectively referred to as "the financials," are the balance sheet, statement of cash flows, and the income statement. The primary financial statement that leaders need to understand and interpret is the income statement, sometimes referred to as the statement of operations, and commonly known as the profit and loss statement or "P&L." The balance sheet and statement of cash flows are primarily used by financial leaders and will be briefly defined.

BALANCE SHEET

The **balance sheet** indicates the financial position of a business enterprise at a particular point in time. It typically represents financial performance at the

BOX 4.1

BASIC ACCOUNTING EQUATION

Assets = Liabilities + Net assets (Owner's equity)

EXHIBIT 4.1

BALANCE SHEET (REGIONAL HEALTH SYSTEM, FY 20X2)

ASSETS		LIABILITIES AND NET ASSETS	
Current assets	$37,477,916	Liabilities	
Fixed assets	$99,523,823	Current liabilities	$57,433,940
Investments	$244,101,733	Long-term liabilities	$81,950,624
		Total liabilities	$139,384,564
		Net assets (fund balance)	$231,866,348
Total assets	$381,103,472	Total liabilities and net assets	$371,250,912

end of an accounting period or fiscal year, but it can also be used for interim accounting periods, such as a month or a quarter. The **basic accounting equation** (Box 4.1) includes the primary components presented in the simple balance sheet shown in Exhibit 4.1.

On the left side of the balance sheet and basic accounting equation is assets that include current and fixed assets and investments. **Current assets**, also referred to as short-term or near-term assets, are usually cash or will become cash within a year. **Fixed assets** are an organization's property, plant, and equipment. **Investments** are typically securities the organization purchases as a long-term investment. The right side of the balance sheet includes liabilities and net assets. **Liabilities** are the organization's obligations to pay someone. Current or short-term liabilities are typically due within 1 year, whereas obligations due longer than 1 year are long-term liabilities. **Net assets** represent the value the organization has to its owners and are the proportion of the assets left over after all liabilities have been paid.

STATEMENT OF CASH FLOWS

The next key financial statement is the **statement of cash flows** that reports where cash resources came from and how they were used during the accounting

EXHIBIT 4.2

STATEMENT OF CASH FLOWS (REGIONAL HEALTH SYSTEM, FY 20X2)

Cash flows from operating activities	
Collections	$ 208,948,281
Payments to suppliers	$ (30,394,522)
Payments to employees	$ (101,315,073)
Net cash from operating activities	$ 77,238,686
Cash flow from investing activities	
Purchase of new equipment	$ (1,532,455)
Net cash used for investing activities	$ (1,532,455)
Cash flow from financing activities	
Borrowing from creditors	$ 31,163,809
Debt payment	$ (17,615,505)
Net cash from financing activities	$ 13,548,304
Net increase/(decrease) in cash	$ 1,566,455
Cash, beginning of year	$ 895,275

period according to operating, investing, or financing activities, shown in Exhibit 4.2. The statement of cash flows is concerned with viability or if the organization can generate enough cash to meet both short- and long-term obligations. The balance sheet shows how much cash the organization has at the end of the accounting period that can be compared year-over-year to see how much the cash balance has changed. However, it doesn't relate how or why it changed. Cash flow from operations is an important focus because it provides information on whether the routine operating activities, such as treating patients, are generating enough cash to cover the organization's obligations to pay its employees and creditors.

INCOME STATEMENT

The last financial statement is the **income statement,** also known as the **operating statement** or activity statement, and commonly referred to as the "P&L." The income statement compares an organization's revenues to its expenses. The financial information contained in the income statement follows the same format and major components as presented in Chapter 2 on how money flows

EXHIBIT 4.3

INCOME STATEMENT (REGIONAL HEALTH SYSTEM, FY 20X2)

Inpatient revenue	$ 295,211,498
Outpatient revenue	$ 349,532,119
Gross revenue ①	$ 644,743,617
Allowances and discounts ②	$ (435,795,336)
Net revenue	$ 208,948,281
Other non-operating revenue ③	$ 1,986,295
Total net revenue	$ 210,934,576
Depreciation expense ④	$ (13,318,450)
Other expenses ⑤	$ (189,311,696)
Total operating expenses	$ (202,630,146)
Net income ⑥	$ 8,304,430

through the healthcare provider organization and also Chapter 3 in developing the operating budget.

The sample income statement, shown in Exhibit 4.3 is used to manage the operations and is therefore one of the most important and commonly used statements for leaders. The income statement is different from the balance sheet, which is a snapshot in time, in that it tells what happened to the organization over a period of time, such as a month, quarter, or year. The income statement shows the revenues received in exchange for the delivery of services and the expenses incurred to generate revenues. It is generally compared to budget goals from a previous period, such as the last month or the same period a year ago. It will be useful to walk through the major components of the income statement.

① Gross Revenue

Gross revenue includes all revenue from patient activities, both inpatient (hospital admission) and outpatient. As presented in Chapter 2, gross charges are the billed amount prior to subtracting any contractual allowances.

② Allowances and Discounts

Deductions from gross revenue, including the private insurance payer contractual allowances, discounts, and charity care.

③ Other Non-Operating Revenue

Revenue received from non-patient activities, such as investments, endowments, gift shop, cafeteria, and parking.

④ Depreciation Expense

Fixed costs from depreciating the value of property, plant, and equipment over their useful life. The amount shown is for the specified period, such as the fiscal year, versus the accumulated (cumulative) depreciation listed on the balance sheet.

⑤ Operating Expenses

These are expenses related to patient care including salaries, wages, benefits, supplies, purchased services, insurance, and the provision or write-off for bad debt. Bad debt is the term used to describe the allowance or amount expected to be paid by the patient or other payer that is determined as uncollectable and is therefore written-off as an expense.

⑥ Net Income

This is the excess revenue over expenses, or the amount of profit realized from the business enterprise's operations after taking out operating expenses, such as labor and supplies.

FINANCIAL RATIO ANALYSIS

The second method for assessing the financial condition of the business enterprise is the **financial ratio analysis**. Financial ratio analysis is a common technique used in both financial statement and operating indicator analyses, covered later in this chapter. It combines values from the financial statements and elsewhere to create single numbers that have easily interpretable economic significance. There are four categories of ratio analyses, listed in Box 4.2 that will be addressed in detail.

Financial ratio analysis facilitates meaningful comparisons given that a single ratio value has little comparative value. In other words, a single number in and of itself is relatively meaningless without comparing it to itself over time or compared to other similar organizations. Two techniques help us interpret financial data: **trend analysis** (time series) and **comparative analysis** (cross-sectional). Figure 4.1 shows Regional Health System's (RHS's) operating revenue and expense over the 3-year analysis period from FY 20X0 to FY 20X2. Figure 4.2 compares RHS's revenue and expense to its market peers in FY 20X2.

> **BOX 4.2**
>
> **FINANCIAL RATIO ANALYSIS CATEGORIES**
> 1. Profitability
> 2. Liquidity
> 3. Asset management
> 4. Debt management

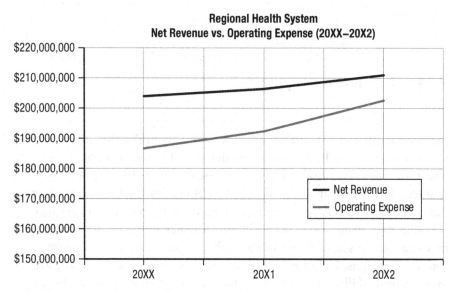

FIGURE 4.1 Time series analysis.

Profitability

Presented in Chapter 2, profitability assesses if the business enterprise is generating sufficient profits to achieve its goals and measures the overall impact of operating decisions on the business's financial condition. Because businesses require profits to remain viable in the long run, profitability ratios are an important measure of financial condition. All profitability ratios require some definition of profit, such as profit per dollar of assets or profit per dollar of revenue.

There are many (perhaps too many) ways to measure profit in healthcare. For example, profit measured on a total basis includes income, such as contributions from sources other than operations. Profit can also be defined by

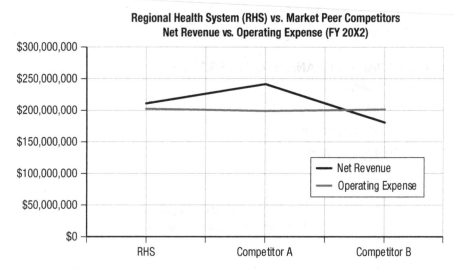

FIGURE 4.2 Cross-sectional analysis.

the revenue that stems solely from operations, typically through providing patient care services. Profit can also be defined either before or after taxes, for investor-owned organizations, and either before or after financial costs, such as interest expense. Finally, profit can be defined on the basis of accounting rules, like net income, or it can be defined as cash flow, such as net income plus non-cash expenses. It would be much easier if one or two profitability ratios gave leaders all of the information they needed for conducting a financial condition analysis. Unfortunately, that is not the case, so we have to consider multiple profitability ratios. Profitability ratios are generally expressed as a percentage rather than in decimal form. Among the many profitability ratios used in healthcare the two most common and important for assessing the financial health of the business enterprise are total margin and operating margin.

Total Margin

Total margin measures profitability as a percentage of total revenues. It measures the ability of a business enterprise to control expenses. For example, a total margin of 5% means that each dollar of total revenues generates five cents in profits. The higher the total margin the better. Total margin includes both operating and non-operating revenue, so a business enterprise could operate at a loss and still show a positive operating margin if non-operating revenue was large enough. Total margin is calculated by dividing total revenue by net income multiplied by 100 to get a percentage, as shown in Box 4.3.

BOX 4.3

CALCULATING TOTAL MARGIN

$$\text{Total margin} = \frac{\text{Net income}}{\text{Total revenue}} \times 100$$

Operating Margin

Presented in Chapter 2, **operating margin** is the most common and important measure of profitability expressed as a percentage of operating revenue. In other words, an operating margin of 3% means that each dollar of operating revenue generates three cents in profit. A higher operating margin indicates higher profitability. Operating expense in the calculation may include both variable and fixed costs, versus **contribution margin**, which is calculated by subtracting only the variable costs from operating revenue. Operating margin is similar to the total margin but focuses on core operations by removing the influence of non-operating revenue. Operating margin is a better measure of the sustainable profitability of the organization because it focuses on business income as opposed to income from other, presumably less dependable sources. Recall the formula for calculating operating margin presented in Box 4.4.

BOX 4.4

CALCULATING OPERATING MARGIN

$$\text{Operating margin} = \frac{\text{Operating revenue} - \text{Operating expense}}{\text{Operating revenue}} \times 100$$

Liquidity Ratio

Liquidity ratios assess if the business enterprise can meet its short-term or cash obligations as they become due. Failure to meet these obligations can lead to financial distress and eventual bankruptcy. In general, creditors prefer a business to be highly liquid or have a large amount of cash and short-term investments. A common liquidity test is **days cash on hand** that measures the number of days that the business enterprise could continue to pay its average daily cash obligations without any new cash resources. Higher values imply higher liquidity and hence are viewed favorably by creditors or those who loan money to the business enterprise. However, business enterprises should not hold excess amounts of cash and short-term investments because these typically provide a lower financial return than long-term investments. Days cash on hand is calculated by cash and near-cash divided by daily cash expenses, shown in Box 4.5.

BOX 4.5

CALCULATING DAYS CASH ON HAND

$$\text{Days cash on hand} = \frac{\text{Cash + Short-term investments}}{\text{(Total expense − Depreciation)}} / 365$$

Asset Management

Asset management ratios assess if the business enterprise has the right amount of assets or resources and measures how efficiently it is using those assets for the volume of services it provides. In other words, a business enterprise that is under-producing or over-producing services may be incurring unnecessary waste and expense. A business that has too many assets for its level of activity or volume is bearing unnecessary costs, while a business enterprise that has too few assets may not be able to respond to potential increased volume and runs the risk of future business disruption.

Total Asset Turnover

A common measure of asset management is total asset turnover. The **total asset turnover ratio** measures the dollars of total revenue per dollar of total assets and is calculated using the formula shown in Box 4.6.

BOX 4.6

CALCULATING TOTAL ASSET TURNOVER RATIO

$$\text{Total asset turnover} = \frac{\text{Total revenue}}{\text{Total assets}}$$

A total asset turnover of two, for example, indicates that each dollar invested in total assets generates two dollars in total revenue. The higher the total asset turnover the more efficient the business enterprise's investment in total assets. Different sub-sectors within the healthcare industry have different capital intensities, or the amount of fixed assets required. For example, hospitals require a large amount of fixed assets and therefore have higher total assets.

Home health businesses typically do not and would therefore have a relatively higher total asset turnover ratio than hospitals.

Inventory Turnover

Another useful asset management ratio is **inventory turnover**. As presented in Box 4.7, inventory turnover measures the dollars of total revenue generated by each dollar of inventory. A higher inventory turnover ratio is better and indicates more efficient use of the business enterprise's inventory.

BOX 4.7

CALCULATING TOTAL INVENTORY TURNOVER RATIO

$$\text{Inventory turnover} = \frac{\text{Total revenue}}{\text{Inventory}}$$

Debt Management (Capital Structure Ratios)

These types of ratios assess if the business is using the right mix of debt and equity. They addresses the amount of debt financing used and are important to understand how the organization is leveraging or can leverage both the risk and the profitability of debt financing. These types of ratios are primarily used by strategic financial leaders.

OPERATING INDICATOR ANALYSIS

Leaders who understand the underlying operating conditions of their business enterprise can better address current and potential financial issues that may impact accomplishing the healthcare provider organization's strategic goals. **Operating indicators** involve the use of specific data primarily from the organization's managerial accounting system to assess financial condition, rather than from the financial statements previously covered. Operating indicators, like the instruments of an airplane, inform a leader what and how they are doing compared to the goals. There are several categories of operating indicators focusing on specific aspects of the business enterprise's operations, listed in Box 4.8.

Profitability

Profitability ratios help explain the profitability assessment made in the financial ratio analysis. Two useful profitability indicators are profit per inpatient discharge and profit per outpatient visit.

BOX 4.8

COMMON OPERATING INDICATORS
1. Profitability
2. Price
3. Volume
4. Length of stay
5. Intensity of service
6. Efficiency
7. Input cost

Profit per Discharge

Profit per discharge measures the amount of profit or the contribution to net income earned on each inpatient discharge. It is calculated by taking inpatient revenue minus inpatient operating expenses divided by total discharges, as shown in Box 4.9. A low or negative value is typically caused by high costs or low reimbursement.

BOX 4.9

CALCULATING PROFIT PER DISCHARGE

$$\text{Profit per discharge} = \frac{\text{Inpatient revenue} - \text{Inpatient operating expenses}}{\text{Total discharges}}$$

Similar to profit per discharge, profit per outpatient visit is calculated using outpatient operating revenue and expense, presented in Box 4.10.

BOX 4.10

CALCULATING PROFIT PER OUTPATIENT VISIT

$$\text{Profit per clinic visit} = \frac{\text{Outpatient revenue} - \text{Outpatient visit operating expense}}{\text{Total outpatient visits}}$$

Price Indicators

Price indicators measure the net revenue received and reflect the deducted contractual allowances. They measure the market's assessment of the value of the services provided versus the healthcare provider organization's assigned value in its pricing schedule. A common measure is net price per inpatient discharge, calculated by dividing net inpatient revenue by total discharges, shown in Box 4.11.

BOX 4.11

CALCULATING NET PRICE PER DISCHARGE

$$\text{Net price per discharge} = \frac{\text{Net inpatient revenue}}{\text{Total discharges}}$$

Volume Indicators

A large proportion of a healthcare provider organization's costs are fixed. Therefore, volume is an important determinant of profitability. Typically, more volume means higher profitability. Among the common inpatient **volume indicators** are average daily census (ADC) and occupancy rate.

Average Daily Census

Also referred to as the census, **ADC** measures inpatient volume based on the number of patients or occupied beds. It is the number of registered and admitted patients at a certain time each day, typically midnight local time. Usually a higher ADC is better because the expected revenue spreads fixed costs over a greater number of patients and therefore increases profitability. A valid interpretation of this measure requires comparison with the number of licensed or staffed beds. Licensed beds are the maximum number of beds that the healthcare provider organization can fill, according to the licensure authority, such as the state. The number of staffed beds or the total possible beds is the number of beds that the organization can fill or patients that it can accommodate due to staffing restrictions. ADC is calculated by dividing the total annual patient days by 365, as shown in Box 4.12.

BOX 4.12

CALCULATING AVERAGE DAILY CENSUS

$$\text{Average daily census} = \frac{\text{Total annual patient days}}{365 \text{ days}}$$

Occupancy Rate

Occupancy rate or occupancy measures inpatient volume as a percentage of the number of beds. As with ADC, the higher the occupancy rate the better, unless it is so high that the healthcare provider organization doesn't have enough capacity to address emergency situations which can also lead to employee burnout and involuntary turnover. To raise the occupancy rate hospitals can increase admissions, increase the length of stay (LOS) which may not be sensible under many reimbursement schemes, or decrease the number of beds. The occupancy rate is calculated as the total annual patient days divided by number of beds multiplied by 365, shown in Box 4.13.

BOX 4.13

CALCULATING OCCUPANCY RATE

$$\text{Occupancy rate} = \frac{\text{Total annual patient days} \times 100}{\text{Number of beds} \times 365}$$

Length of Stay Indicators

A large proportion of a healthcare provider organization's inpatient reimbursement is based on admissions and the type of diagnosis. Therefore, LOS can have a significant impact on profitability, both favorably and unfavorably. Two common **LOS indicators** are LOS and adjusted LOS.

Length of Stay

LOS is an efficiency indicator measuring the number of days that a patient stays in the hospital. A shorter LOS is typically better and means relatively lower total cost of care. However, financial penalties may be assessed for Medicare patients with certain diagnoses who are discharged too soon and are readmitted to a hospital within a certain period. It is calculated as the total annual patient days divided by total inpatient discharges, shown in Box 4.14.

BOX 4.14

CALCULATING LENGTH OF STAY

$$\text{Length of stay} = \frac{\text{Total annual patient days}}{\text{Total discharges}}$$

Adjusted Length of Stay

Adjusted LOS accounts for the patient mix or how sick the patient is, also known as acuity. This measure is similar to LOS except that it adjusts for the fact that hospitals differ greatly in the inpatient complexity of care they deliver. Hospitals with a higher acuity treat more complex diagnoses and hence would be expected to have a longer adjusted LOS. Adjusted LOS removes any potential bias created by differences in case mix. Adjusted LOS is calculated by the total annual patient days divided by total inpatient discharges multiplied by the case mix index (CMI), shown in Box 4.15.

BOX 4.15

CALCULATING ADJUSTED LENGTH OF STAY

$$\text{Adjusted LOS} = \frac{\text{Total annual patient days}}{\text{Total discharges} \times \text{CMI}}$$

Intensity of Service Indicators

The costs of providing services and the associated revenues are a function of the intensity of the services provided. Common **intensity of service indicators** include CMI, cost per inpatient discharge, and cost per outpatient visit.

Case Mix Index

CMI measures the average relative weight and summation of all of the hospital's **Medicare severity-diagnosis related group** (MS-DRG) inpatient discharges. Inpatients are assigned a unique and specific MS-DRG based on their clinical determination of diagnosis. For example, MS-DRG 470 is for major joint replacement or reattachment of lower extremity without major complications. The CMI reflects the diversity, complexity, and resource needs of all the patients in a hospital. Higher CMI equates to more reimbursement, based on documentation and coding accuracy. Although the MS-DRG weights provided by the Centers for Medicare & Medicaid (CMS) were designed for the Medicare population, they are applied to all discharges regardless of the payer.

Cost per Discharge or Outpatient Visit

Cost per inpatient discharge or outpatient visit measures the average cost of each inpatient stay or outpatient visit. Lower costs equate to higher profitability. As shown in Box 4.16, cost per discharge is calculated by taking the total inpatient operating expense divided by total inpatient discharges. Note that the cost per outpatient visit can be calculated using total outpatient operating expense and total (outpatient) visits instead of the inpatient equivalent.

BOX 4.16

CALCULATING COST PER DISCHARGE OR OUTPATIENT VISIT

Cost per discharge = $\dfrac{\text{Total inpatient operating expense}}{\text{Total discharges}}$

Efficiency Indicators

Efficiency indicators measure the amount of resources used to provide services or the amount of inputs needed. As previously discussed, labor is a key input in delivering healthcare services and therefore often the primary focus of efficiency indicators. In general, the more efficiently the services are being provided, the greater the profitability. Note that several of these indicators use **full-time equivalents (FTE)** to measure the amount of labor used. FTEs convert part-time employees into full-time employees. FTE calculations are addressed in more detail in Chapter 6. Common efficiency indicators include FTEs per occupied bed and hours per inpatient discharge or outpatient hours per outpatient visit.

FTEs per Occupied Bed

FTEs per occupied bed measures the productivity of labor devoted to inpatient services as a function of the number of patients. Because the provision of inpatient services is labor intensive, labor productivity plays an important role in inpatient costs. In addition to the number of patients, the intensity of services provided also affects the requirement for labor resources. Thus, this ratio often is adjusted for case mix differentials by multiplying the denominator by the all-patient CMI. The FTEs per occupied bed is calculated by taking the inpatient FTEs divided by total annual patient days divided by 365, as presented in Box 4.17.

BOX 4.17

FTES PER OCCUPIED BED

FTEs per occupied bed = $\dfrac{\text{Inpatient FTEs}}{\text{Total annual patient days}/365}$ = $\dfrac{\text{Inpatient FTEs}}{\text{ADC}}$

Total Employee Hours per Discharge or Outpatient Visit

Total hours per discharge measures the productivity of labor devoted to inpatient (or outpatient) services and uses discharges (or visits) rather than ADC and labor hours as input. This is calculated by taking the inpatient FTEs multiplied by 2,080 total annual paid hours all divided by total inpatient discharges, as shown in Box 4.18.

BOX 4.18

TOTAL EMPLOYEE HOURS PER DISCHARGE OR OUTPATIENT VISIT

$$\text{Hours per discharge} = \frac{\text{Inpatient (or outpatient) FTEs} \times 2{,}080}{\text{Total discharges (or outpatient visits)}}$$

Input Cost Indicators

Input costs indicators are a function of both the quantity of inputs used and the cost per unit of input and focus on the cost of resources, such as labor. Common indicators include salary per FTE, fringe benefits percentage, compensation costs per inpatient discharge, capital costs per inpatient discharge, supply costs per inpatient discharge, and professional liability cost per inpatient discharge. For example, labor costs depend on both the number of FTEs and the wage rates paid per FTE. Efficiency indicators, discussed in the previous section, measure the amount of resources used. The unit cost indicators presented in this section focus on the cost of those resources. In general, the lower the cost of an organization's inputs, the greater its profitability.

Salary per FTE

Salary per FTE measures average labor cost, not including fringe benefits, per employee. Wages are hourly based on time worked and salaries are paid on an annual rate. Because labor is the largest input in the provision of healthcare services, control over these costs is critical to profitability. Note that wages generally describe the pay of workers paid on the basis of their time worked, such as hourly, daily, weekly. Salaries are typically paid for higher-level employees, such as managers, who are compensated at an annual rate regardless of the amount of time they work. This ratio is often adjusted for wage rate differentials by multiplying the denominator by the wage index. As shown in Box 4.19, salary per FTE is the total salary and wage expense divided by total FTEs.

BOX 4.19

CALCULATING SALARY PER FTE

Salary per FTE = $\dfrac{\text{Salary and wage expense}}{\text{Total FTEs}}$

ADJUSTED CALCULATIONS

There is often the need to "adjust" calculations to account for the need to aggregate measures that incorporate and equate both inpatient and outpatient volume. This allows for more accurate productivity measurement and resource planning. Representative adjusted measures include admissions, ADC, and patient days. There is also the need to reflect adjusting for the acuity level by adjusting the case mix. This reflects and adjusts for the relatively higher expected use of resources for sicker patients, especially when accounting for labor productivity and use of services and supplies that can affect the total cost of care. The most common case mix-adjusted (CMA) calculations are for discharges, LOS, volume, revenue, and expense.

Adjusted Admissions

Adjusted admissions (AA) is an aggregate measure of workload reflecting the number of patients admitted during the reporting period, plus an estimate of the volume of outpatient services, expressed in units equivalent to an inpatient day in terms of the level of effort. The figure is derived by first multiplying the number of outpatient visits by the ratio of outpatient revenue per outpatient visit to inpatient revenue per inpatient day. The product, which represents the number of admissions attributable to outpatient services, is then added to the number of admissions. The purpose of this calculation is to summarize overall productivity and calculate a unit cost that would include both inpatient and outpatient admissions. Most any financial or operating measure can be adjusted for case mix. The most common are LOS, volume, revenue, and expense.

Adjusted Average Daily Census

Adjusted ADC is an estimate of the average number of patients, both inpatients and outpatients, receiving care each day during the reporting period, which is usually 12 months. It is calculated by dividing the number of inpatient day equivalents, also called adjusted inpatient days, by the number of days in the reporting period.

Adjusted Patient Days

Adjusted patient days is an aggregate figure reflecting the number of days of inpatient care plus an estimate of the volume of outpatient services expressed in units equivalent to an inpatient day in terms of level of effort. It is derived by first multiplying the number of outpatient visits by the ratio of outpatient revenue per outpatient visit to inpatient revenue per inpatient day. The product, which represents the number of patient days attributable to outpatient services, is then added to the number of inpatient days. The purpose of this calculation is to summarize overall productivity and calculate a unit cost that would include both inpatient and outpatient activities. Adjusted patient days is calculated by taking the inpatient days divided by the percentage of inpatient revenues to total patient revenues.

Case Mix-Adjusted Calculations

The CMA discharge, for example, is for adjusting the average cost per discharge relative to the adjusted average cost for other hospitals by dividing the average cost per discharge by the CMI. The adjusted average cost per discharge would reflect the charges reported for the types of cases treated in a given year. For example, if the average cost per patient of $1,000 with a CMI of 0.80 for a given year, the adjusted cost per patient is $1,000 divided by 0.80, which is $1,250. Likewise, if a peer comparison hospital has an average cost per patient of $1,500 and a CMI of 1.25, its adjusted cost per patient is $1,500 divided by 1.25 or $1,200. If a hospital has a CMI greater than 1.00, its adjusted cost per patient or per day will be lower. Conversely, if a hospital has a CMI less than 1.00, its adjusted cost will be higher.

REGIONAL HEALTH SYSTEM CASE EXAMPLE: CONDUCTING A FINANCIAL CONDITION ANALYSIS

Due to continued financial and operating challenges straining already thin operating margins, the CEO has engaged a task force comprised of key internal stakeholders and external expertise to conduct and present a comprehensive financial condition analysis to identify and assess opportunities for improving financial performance without compromising quality. Using the guidance and information provided in the chapter, the data contained within the financial statements (income statement), and the selected measures of financial performance contained in the Chapter 4 spreadsheet (visit connect.springerpub.com/content/book/978-0-8261-4464-5/chapter/ch04 and access the show chapter supplementary dropdown at the beginning of the chapter), the task force conducts the financial forensic analysis to identify financial and operating trends and consider potential opportunities for improvement. Approaches and specific actions for reducing expense and increasing revenue will be addressed later in Chapters 6, 7, and 8. The specific financial statements, financial ratios, and operating indicators assessed between the 3-year period from FY 20XX to FY 20X2 includes:

1. Financial statements.
   - Income statement (total operating revenue, total operating expenses, net income)

2. Financial ratio analysis
   - Profitability (operating margin)
   - Liquidity (days cash on hand)
   - Asset management (total asset turnover)

3. Operating indicator analysis
   - Profitability (profit per discharge)
   - Price (net price per discharge)
   - Volume (discharges, occupancy rate, ADC)
   - LOS (CMA LOS)
   - Intensity of service (CMI)
   - Efficiency (FTEs per occupied bed, paid hours per discharge)
   - Input cost (cost per discharge)

The interpretation of the available financial and operating data (both favorable and unfavorable) and the potential opportunities for improving financial performance are presented in Table 4.1. The source data used for all of the financial condition analysis calculations are provided on Springer Connect (visit connect.springerpub.com/content/book/978-0-8261-4464-5/chapter/ch04 and access the show chapter supplementary dropdown at the beginning of the chapter). These data will be used for other financial calculations referenced throughout the text.

CATEGORY	INDICATORS	FINANCIAL CONDITION ANALYSIS	POTENTIAL OPPORTUNITIES
Income statement	Profitability	RHS experienced relatively flat operating revenue and increasing expenses. **Net revenue** increased by $6.9 million (3.3%); however, **operating expenses** increased at a faster rate, almost $16 million (7.9%). **Net income** decreased $9 million (109%).	Both soft volume and increasing operating expense trends present an opportunity to assess and prioritize a comprehensive yet focused plan to improve and sustain operating margin.
Financial ratio analysis	Profitability	**Operating margin** decreased 8.2% to 3.3% (151%).	Assess cash needs versus potential to invest with higher return.
	Liquidity	**Days cash on hand** increased 1.4 days from 3.3 days in FY 20X0 to 4.7 days in 20X2.	
	Asset management	Total asset turnover increased 8.8% to 0.67.	Trending favorably with additional opportunity to increase throughput
Operating indicator analysis	Profitability	**Profit per discharge** (contribution to net income) decreased $338 (197%) from $511 to $172.	Examine potential opportunities for reducing operating expense reduction.
	Price	**Net price per discharge** decreased $927 (16.9%)	Assess fee schedule, negotiated reimbursement, and patient collections.
	Volume	Inpatient **discharge** volume decreased 2,296 (16.4%); however, patient days were relatively flat and down only 0.95%. **Occupancy rate** remained steady, down only 0.7%. **Average daily census** decreased steadily, down 13.3 days (8.1%).	Potential opportunities to increase volume through covered Medicare preventive testing services. Assess growth opportunities in high-margin services.
	Length of stay	**Case mix-adjusted LOS** increased 0.35 days (10.8%).	Increasing LOS and decreasing CMI present an opportunity to assess care processes to reduce unwarranted clinical variation.
	Intensity of service	**CMI** decreased 0.08 (6.2).	
	Efficiency	**FTEs per occupied bed** increased gradually 3.9% and 2.7% per year. 0.30 FTE total over the 3-year review period. **Paid hours per discharge** decreased 7.82 hours (7.8%). Salary per FTE increased $2,397 (4.9%).	Increasing operating expenses as a percent of revenue indicates opportunities for aggressive expense control of input costs including labor expense through benchmarking and improved workflow. Also tight management of supplies, implants, and purchased services and their utilization.
	Input cost	RHS's **cost per discharge** decreased $622 (11.3%).	

SUMMARY

Knowing how to interpret financial data and information is a critical leadership skill to support the organization's mission and achieve its strategic goals. Basic financial statements, such as the income statement or P&L, financial ratios, and operating indicators provide valuable insight to identify opportunities to improve financial performance. Conducting a financial condition analysis provides a comprehensive and effective approach to assess and improve financial performance.

CALLS TO ACTION

Leaders should:

- Be familiar with the basic measures of financial and operating performance.
- Recall how to calculate key financial statements, operating indicators, and financial ratios.
- Apply how to interpret key financial statements, operating indicators, and financial ratios to conduct a financial condition analysis.

CHAPTER 5

UNDERSTANDING FINANCIAL AND OPERATING VARIANCE

INTRODUCTION

As discussed in Chapter 3, developing the operating budget is a critical decision-making process that provides the plan for managing the financial and operating performance of the business enterprise. Despite its usefulness as a performance measurement and management tool, the budget cannot always account for unexpected events or trends that affect financial performance, such as soft patient volume, increased labor costs, and unforeseen market forces. When there is a variance between the prescribed goals of the healthcare provider organization and the actual financial and operating performance, leaders are responsible for assessing and diagnosing the root cause or causes to support taking the appropriate, deliberate, and decisive corrective action.

A **variance** is any deviation from a planned target identified in the budget or other guidance compared to actual performance typically published in one or more of the basic financial statements presented in Chapter 4. A financial variance can either be favorable or unfavorable. While it's important to understand the causes of favorable variances to ensure the contributing factors are sustained, variance analysis is primarily focused on unfavorable results and trends. The goal of effective financial and operations management is to prevent, if possible, or to correct unfavorable variances to achieve the desired targets.

Healthcare leaders are not adequately prepared or given access to the right resources to identify and interpret the cause of financial and operating variances, much less develop and implement effective tactics to address them. Leaders with clinical backgrounds especially, despite their extensive training and use of quantitative data, such as patient vitals and lab values, are often ill-prepared and ill-at-ease making sense of financial data and reports. Most physicians, for example, aren't taught basic management skills and receive little if any on-the-job training in the business of medicine.[1] Otherwise competent and qualified clinicians, including nurses and allied health providers, are no exception.

For example, during a meeting with a clinical nurse manager to review her department's monthly financial performance she admitted her lack of understanding about how to interpret the financial data and translate it into the appropriate actions to achieve her budgeted financial targets. "If it's a patient at the bedside, I know exactly what to do, but clinicians are not effectively trained in financial management." The nurse leader's candid comments summarize the common challenge and frustration for many leaders and served as the inspiration for developing a formal and deliberate process to empower healthcare leaders, both clinical and nonclinical, to better understand and manage their business enterprise and support achieving their financial goals through variance analysis.

FROM PATIENT MANAGEMENT TO FINANCIAL MANAGEMENT

The process for diagnosing and treating patients can be related to the process for assessing and improving the financial well-being of a business enterprise. Clinicians are trained to follow prescriptive guidelines for examining and treating a patient, including making the initial diagnosis. This process is based on collecting the patient's history and physical exam results, which may require diagnostic testing, such as labs or imaging studies, before developing the treatment plan and then following-up with the patient to make sure the treatment plan was effective. Beyond the basic process for diagnosing and treating patients, evidence-based guidelines are used to educate and train clinicians on the most effective and efficient approach for treating specific diagnoses or diseases, such as hypertension or diabetes. Algorithmic protocols, commonly referred to as a clinical pathway or integrated care pathway, are characterized by the application of process management thinking to standardize and improve clinical outcomes and patient safety.

A parallel to this clinical example is conducting a financial variance analysis, illustrated in Table 5.1. As discussed in Chapter 3, basic financial statements contain relevant data for a specified period and can be used to identify unfavorable variances. Further analysis can be conducted to uncover the root cause of the variance and then develop, implement, and monitor the appropriate corrective action plan. Similar to a clinical pathway that provides a standard guideline for diagnosing and treating a patient, a **financial pathway** provides a best-practice framework and step-by-step process for analyzing financial and operations data to identify and interpret variances with the ultimate goal of taking the appropriate corrective action to improve financial performance.

TABLE 5.1 Clinical Assessment and Financial Analysis Parallel

STEP	PATIENT MANAGEMENT	FINANCIAL MANAGEMENT
1	Conduct the initial triage and diagnose the patient's problem	Conduct the initial review of basic financial statements and data to identify and prioritize variances
2	Conduct diagnostic testing to validate assumptions (lab, radiology)	Collect and analyze supporting documents (invoices, time reports)
3	Develop and communicate the treatment plan	Develop and implement the corrective action plan
4	Follow-up and modify the treatment plan as needed to achieve the desired clinical outcome	Continuously measure, monitor, and manage as needed to achieve the budget target

VARIANCE ANALYSIS

Discussed in Chapter 4, the profit and loss (P&L) statement provides a snapshot of a business enterprise's financial performance compared to budgeted goals. It typically includes the prior month and prior year for comparison. Year-to-year comparisons allow for identifying volume, revenue, and expense variances due to seasonal trends, also known as seasonality. **Seasonality** is anticipated fluctuations in volume due to recurring external events or trends, such as higher patient volume during flu season. The P&L statement should include calculated variances. If not, they must be calculated as shown in Table 5.2, where the "Actual" amounts are subtracted from the "Budget" amounts to calculate the "Variance" column.

Variances can be classified as favorable or unfavorable. A negative variance is not always unfavorable. Whether the variance is favorable or unfavorable depends on if the amount is positive or negative and also if it is a revenue or expense. As discussed in Chapter 2, a negative variance can be favorable or unfavorable and can be presented with a minus sign, brackets or parentheses, in red, or a combination of all three. Table 5.3 provides a guide to identifying the type of variance.

Table 5.4 provides an example of how to determine if the variance is positive or negative and if it is under budget or over budget. **Under budget** refers to exceeding the targeted revenue or expense, while **over budget** means that the target was missed or exceeded. In the example, total revenue is $500 over budget meaning the actual revenue collected for the period was $500 more than the budget target. The total expense for the period was $1,000 over budget. In other words, more money was spent on operating expense than planned. Therefore, even though the business enterprise had a $500 positive net income or profit, the variance was unfavorable because it was $1,000 under budget. The variance percentages are calculated by dividing the "Variance" by the "Actual" amount.

TABLE 5.2 **Calculating Financial Variance Example**

COMPONENT	BUDGET	ACTUAL	VARIANCE
Revenue	$10,000	$9,500	($500)
Expense	$8,500	$7,500	$1,000
Net income	$1,500	$2,000	$500

TABLE 5.3 **Favorable or Unfavorable Variance**

COMPONENT	POSITIVE (+)	TYPE	NEGATIVE (−)	TYPE
Revenue	Favorable	Over budget	Unfavorable	Under budget
Expense	Unfavorable	Under budget	Favorable	Over budget

TABLE 5.4 **Calculating Financial Variance**

| COMPONENT | BUDGET | ACTUAL | VARIANCE | | TYPE |
			AMOUNT	PERCENT	
Revenue	$10,000	$10,500	$500	4.8%	Favorable, over budget
Expense	$8,500	$10,000	($1,500)	15.0%	Unfavorable, over budget
Net income	$1,500	$500	($1,000)	200.0%	Unfavorable, under budget

TABLE 5.5 **Process to Identify Unfavorable Variances**

Step 1	Identify net operating income variance
Step 2	Calculate operating revenue variance
Step 2A	Identify volume variance
Step 3	Identify operating expense variance
Step 3A	Identify labor expense variance
Step 3B	Identify non-labor expense variance
Step 4	Examine variance root cause
Step 5	Develop and implement corrective action plan

FINANCIAL PATHWAY

The financial pathway provided in Figure 5.1 and also in Appendix C is a logical step-by-step process for leaders with accountability for a business enterprise to identify, prioritize, and manage unfavorable variances to achieve financial and operations performance goals. Specific **variance thresholds**, or financial controls, expressed in terms of both dollars and percentages should be established by senior leaders during the budgeting process. The step-by-step process for identifying unfavorable variances is provided in Table 5.5 and explored using the financial pathway provided in the following case example.

REGIONAL HEALTH SYSTEM CASE EXAMPLE: VARIANCE ANALYSIS FOR THE DEPARTMENT OF SURGICAL SERVICES

Due to continued financial challenges straining already thin hospital operating margins, the Regional Health System's (RHS's) CEO implemented a department-level monthly operations review (MOR) using the agenda in Box 5.1. The purpose and goals of the MOR are: to provide a framework for promoting accountability to improve financial and operations performance that achieves budget goals; to identify and provide the necessary resources for success, such as improved financial management "know how" among leaders; and to provide timely, accurate, and actionable financial and operations information for leaders to support improved decision-making. A sample reference MOR meeting agenda is presented in Box 5.1. The premise of introducing the MOR is for leaders to assess variance from their operating budget and to present their corrective action plans to support achieving the healthcare provider organization's financial goals.

BOX 5.1

MONTHLY OPERATIONS REVIEW AGENDA

1. Review purpose and goals of the MOR
2. Review financial and operating statistics:
   - Profit and loss statement
   - Salaries and wages expense
   - Supply expense
   - Purchased services expense
   - Weekly labor productivity report
   - Open position report
3. Review financial and operating thresholds (MOR Financial Pathway)
4. Review variance action plan
5. Discussion and next steps

Almost 40% of the healthcare provider organization's total net income variance to budget fiscal year-to-date is attributed to surgical services. Beyond the CEOs guidance, the RHS CFO has asked the Director for the Surgical Services to take a "deep dive" into the department's financial and operating performance to identify the causes for missing the budget targets and then to devise and implement an appropriate action plan to get back on track within the next quarter. Using the financial pathway and established thresholds in Figure 5.1 and the financial data from the monthly P&L statement in Appendix D from RHS's Department of Surgical Services, the director conducted a variance analysis using the financial pathway illustrated in the case example.

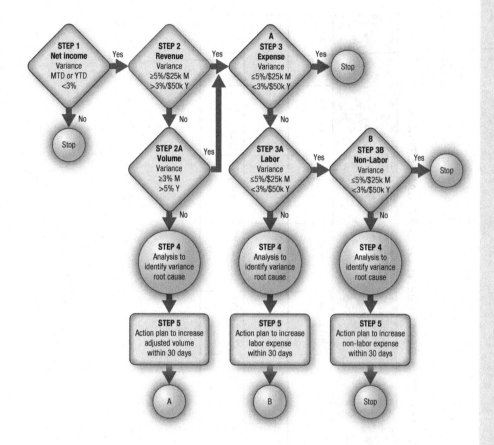

FIGURE 5.1 Financial pathway for Regional Health System's Department of Surgical Services.
M, month; MTD, month-to-date; Y, year; YTD, year-to-date.

STEP 1. Determining Net Income Variance

Beginning at a high level of analysis, the first step shown in Figure 5.2 is to determine net income from operations. Recall from Chapter 2 that net income is calculated by subtracting operating expenses from operating revenue.

Surgical Services

The net income variance threshold for the department is 3%, both for the month and year-to-date. Therefore, the −4.6% for the month and −4.1% for the year are unfavorable variances that require further review and analysis to determine the cause so the appropriate corrective action plan can be developed and implemented (see Exhibit 5.1). Action planning to manage and reduce variances is covered later in the chapter.

EXHIBIT 5.1

NET INCOME VARIANCE FOR REGIONAL HEALTH SYSTEM'S DEPARTMENT OF SURGICAL SERVICES

	SEPTEMBER (FY 20X2)				FY 20X2 YEAR-TO-DATE			
	PRIOR YEAR ACTUAL	BUDGET	ACTUAL	VARIANCE	VARIANCE PERCENT	PRIOR YEAR ACTUAL	BUDGET	ACTUAL	VARIANCE	VARIANCE PERCENT
Total Operating Revenue	$1,379,720	$1,332,583	$1,360,132	$27,549	2.0%	$4,139,160	$12,152,301	$12,006,477	($145,824)	−1.2%
Total Operating Expense	$450,039	$431,934	$498,954	($67,020)	13.4%	$2,792,101	$3,887,406	$4,066,003	($178,597)	4.4%
Net Income/ (Loss)	$929,681	$900,649	$861,178	($39,471)	−4.6%	$1,347,059	$8,264,895	$7,940,474	($324,421)	−4.1%

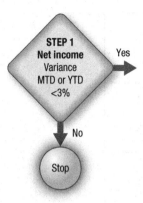

FIGURE 5.2 Step 1: Determining net income variance.
MTD, month-to-date; YTD, year-to-date.

STEP 2. Determining Operating Revenue Variance

The next step, shown in Figure 5.3, is to determine if there is any unfavorable operating revenue variance. If there is an unfavorable variance, is it due to lower than anticipated patient volume? The department revenue amount threshold that triggers the need for further analysis is less than or equal to 5% or $25,000 of the budget target for the month (M) and less than or equal to 3% or $50,000 for the year-to-date (Y). Given the financial data from the department P&L statement shown in Exhibit 5.2, monthly revenue exceeds the budgeted target and therefore does not require explanation. However, year-to-date

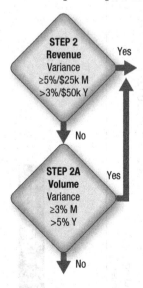

FIGURE 5.3 Step 2: Determining operating revenue variance and Step 2A: Determining volume variance.
M, month; Y, year.

EXHIBIT 5.2

TOTAL OPERATING REVENUE VARIANCE FOR REGIONAL HEALTH SYSTEM'S DEPARTMENT OF SURGICAL SERVICES

| | SEPTEMBER (FY 20X2) | | | | | FY 20X2 YEAR-TO-DATE | | | |
	PRIOR YEAR ACTUAL	BUDGET	ACTUAL	VARIANCE	VARIANCE PERCENT	PRIOR YEAR ACTUAL	BUDGET	ACTUAL	VARIANCE	VARIANCE PERCENT
Total Operating Revenue	$1,379,720	$1,332,583	$1,360,132	$27,549	2.0%	$4,139,160	$12,152,301	$12,006,477	($145,824)	−1.2%

EXHIBIT 5.3

VOLUME VARIANCE FOR REGIONAL HEALTH SYSTEM'S DEPARTMENT OF SURGICAL SERVICES

| | SEPTEMBER (FY 20X2) | | | | | FY 20X2 YEAR-TO-DATE | | | |
	PRIOR YEAR ACTUAL	BUDGET	ACTUAL	VARIANCE	VARIANCE PERCENT	PRIOR YEAR ACTUAL	BUDGET	ACTUAL	VARIANCE	VARIANCE PERCENT
Total Units of Service (Adjusted Surgeries)	712	670	699	29	4.1%	2,038	1,916	2,528	612	24.2%

actual operating revenue variance compared to budget is ($145,824), exceeding the dollar threshold and warranting further review and a corrective action plan.

STEP 2A. Determining Volume Variance

A revenue variance can be attributed to one or more factors. Following the financial pathway, the next level of analysis review is to determine if the cause is due to decreased volume, a variable over which a leader can exert influence by ensuring easy access and exemplary service for both patients and referring providers.

The monthly surgical volume is 29 cases or 4.1% more than budgeted for the month, as presented in Exhibit 5.3, which is most likely the cause of the favorable variance and assuming no other change in any other revenue driver, such as payer mix or negotiated rates. Determining the year-to-date cause of the unfavorable variance even though actual volume exceeds budget by 612 cases requires reviewing the variation in previous months to identify and assess volume trends by surgical specialty, by surgeon, and by the type of surgery. Tactics to address soft volume are addressed in Chapter 8.

STEP 3. Determining Operating Expense Variance

The next step, presented in Figure 5.4, is to determine if there is any variance in operating expense. Compared to the variance threshold for department monthly expense of greater than or equal to 5% or $25,000 and greater than or equal to 3% or $50,000 for the year-to-date, there is an unfavorable variance of $67,020 (–13.4%) for the month and an unfavorable variance of $178,597 (–4.4%) year-to-date (shown in Exhibit 5.4). Both variances warrant further analysis to determine the specific cause.

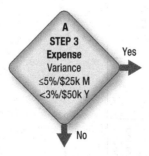

FIGURE 5.4 Step 3: Determining operating expense variance.
M, month; Y, year.

EXHIBIT 5.4

OPERATING EXPENSE VARIANCE FOR REGIONAL HEALTH SYSTEM'S DEPARTMENT OF SURGICAL SERVICES

	SEPTEMBER (FY 20X2)				FY 20X2 YEAR-TO-DATE				
	PRIOR YEAR ACTUAL	BUDGET	ACTUAL	VARIANCE	VARIANCE PERCENT	PRIOR YEAR ACTUAL	BUDGET	ACTUAL	VARIANCE	VARIANCE PERCENT
Total Operating Expense	$450,039	$431,934	$498,954	($67,020)	−13.4%	$2,792,101	$3,887,406	$4,066,003	($178,597)	−4.4%

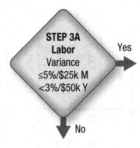

FIGURE 5.5 Step 3A: Determining labor expense variance.
M, month; Y, year.

STEP 3A. Determining Labor Expense Variance (Figure 5.5)

As the single largest operating expense category, labor expense is the most important item for healthcare leaders to understand and aggressively manage to reduce unnecessary expense. The Department of Surgical Services has an unfavorable labor expense variance of $44,502 (–19.9%) for the month and $85,752 (–5%) for the year, as shown in Exhibit 5.5. The labor variance contributes to two thirds of the monthly total operating expense variance and almost half of the year-to-date variance.

Next it is important to conduct additional analyses to understand the specific cause of the labor expense variance, so the corrective action plan targets the right opportunities for improvement. There are three types of labor expense variance: rate, efficiency, and volume. The three variances together explain the entire labor expense variance. In all three variance calculations presented in the following, "Budget" is subtracted from "Actual." This causes negative variances to be favorable and positive variances to be unfavorable, which may be confusing. If this is the case, the calculations can be reversed to subtract "Actual" from "Budget," so the positive variances are favorable and negative variances are unfavorable.

Rate Variance

Labor **rate variance** measures the impact of the labor cost or rate on the department's overall financial performance. Calculating the labor rate variance for the department uses the basic formula provided in Exhibit 5.6 using the data provided in Exhibit 5.7. Applying the formula shows an unfavorable labor rate variance of $23,377, calculated as follows.

EXHIBIT 5.5

LABOR EXPENSE DETAIL FOR REGIONAL HEALTH SYSTEM'S DEPARTMENT OF SURGICAL SERVICES

	SEPTEMBER (FY 20X2)					FY 20X2 YEAR-TO-DATE				
	PRIOR YEAR ACTUAL	BUDGET	ACTUAL	VARIANCE	VARIANCE PERCENT	PRIOR YEAR ACTUAL	BUDGET	ACTUAL	VARIANCE	VARIANCE PERCENT
Labor Expenses										
3010 Director Salary	$8,149	$8,444	$8,444	$0	0.0%	$73,215	$75,996	$75,996	$0	0.0%
3020 RN Salaries & Wages	$172,190	$131,845	$172,190	($40,345)	−23.4%	$516,570	$1,186,605	$1,253,328	($66,723)	−5.3%
3030 LVN Salaries & Wages	$31,238	$27,800	$31,238	($3,438)	−11.0%	$93,714	$250,200	$265,788	($15,588)	−5.9%
3050 Aide Salaries & Wages	$8,712	$7,993	$8,712	($719)	−8.3%	$26,136	$71,937	$76,331	($4,394)	−5.8%
3070 Clerical Salaries & Wages	$3,312	$3,312	$3,312	$0	0.0%	$10,959	$29,808	$28,855	$953	3.3%
Total Labor Expenses	$223,601	$179,394	$223,896	($44,502)	−19.9%	$720,594	$1,614,546	$1,700,298	($85,752)	−5.0%

EXHIBIT 5.6

CALCULATING LABOR RATE VARIANCE

Actual labor cost per hour – budgeted labor cost per hour × total actual labor hours
Actual labor cost – budgeted labor cost × total labor hours

TABLE 5.6 Labor Rate Variance Description

RATE VARIANCE	
Favorable	Labor rate per hour was less than budgeted
Unfavorable	Labor rate per hour was more than budgeted

The rate variance for the department using the data in Exhibit 5.7 is calculated as follows:

$42.24	Actual labor cost per hour
– $37.83	Budgeted labor cost per hour
$4.41	Labor rate variance (actual vs. budgeted cost per hour)
× 5,301 hours	Actual labor hours
$23,377	Rate variance (Unfavorable)

Since the labor rate per hour was more than budgeted, the labor rate variance is unfavorable, as shown in Table 5.6.

Efficiency Variance

Efficiency variance measures the impact of labor hours on the department's financial performance. This measure is used to assess how effectively the department is staffing to meet its volume demands. In order to perform this analysis and calculation to determine the amount of labor expense efficiency variance, the average number of total productive hours to produce a unit of service (UoS) must be determined, such as the number of productive hours per discharge.

Applying the formula provided in Exhibit 5.8 and using the data provided in Exhibit 5.7, the labor efficiency rate variance for the department is calculated as follows:

5,301 hours	Actual labor hours to produce actual UoS $\left\{ \begin{array}{l} \text{Budgeted labor hours} \\ \text{per UoS (7.00)} \times \\ \text{Procedures (699)} \end{array} \right.$
– 4,893 hours	Budgeted labor hours to produce actual UoS
408	Labor usage variance
× $37.83	Budgeted labor rate
$15,435	Efficiency variance (Unfavorable)

EXHIBIT 5.7

MONTHLY LABOR EXPENSE DETAIL FOR REGIONAL HEALTH SYSTEM'S DEPARTMENT OF SURGICAL SERVICES

SEPTEMBER FY 20X2

Labor Expense	Actual	Budget	Variance	% Variance	
Director	$ 8,444	$ 8,444	$ –	0.0%	
RN	$ 172,190	$ 131,845	$ (40,345)	–30.6%	U
LVN	$ 31,238	$ 27,800	$ (3,438)	–12.4%	U
Aide	$ 8,712	$ 7,993	$ (719)	–9.0%	
Clerical	$ 3,312	$ 3,312	$ –	0.0%	
Total Labor Expense	$ 223,896	$ 179,394	$ (44,502)	–24.8%	U
Labor Hours					
Director	160	160	0	0.0%	
RN	3,280	2,848	(432)	–15.2%	U
LVN	1,144	910	(234)	–25.7%	U
Aide	477	584	107	18.3%	
Clerical	240	240	0	0.0%	
Total Labor Hours	5,301	4,742	(559)	–11.8%	U
UoS					
Procedures (adjusted)	699	670	29	4.3%	F
Labor cost per hour	$ 42.24	$ 37.83	(4.41)	–11.7%	U
Labor hours per UoS	7.58	7.00	(0.58)	–8.3%	U

1. Price (or Rate) Variance		
Actual labor cost per hour	$ 42.24	
Budgeted labor cost per hour	$ 37.83	U
Rate variance	$ 4.41	U
Actual labor hours	5,301	
	$ (23,377)	U
2. Efficiency Variance		
Actual labor hours to produce actual UoS	5,301	
Budgeted labor hours to produce actual UoS	4,893	U
Labor usage variance	408	U
Budgeted labor rate	$ 37.83	
	$ 15,435	U
3. Volume Variance		
Budgeted labor hours to produce actual UoS	4,893	F
Budgeted labor hours to produce budgeted UoS	4,742	
Labor volume variance	151	U
Budgeted labor rate	$ 37.83	U
	$ 5,712	U
Total Labor Expense variance	$ 44,524	U

F, favorable variance; U, unfavorable variance; UoS, units of service.

EXHIBIT 5.8

CALCULATING LABOR EFFICIENCY VARIANCE

Actual labor hours to produce actual UoS – Budgeted labor hours to produce actual UoS × Budgeted labor rate

Actual labor cost – Budgeted labor cost × Total labor hours

TABLE 5.7 Labor Efficiency Variance Description

EFFICIENCY VARIANCE	
Favorable	Labor hours per UoS were less than budgeted
Unfavorable	Labor hours per UoS were more than budgeted

UoS, units of service.

Since the labor hours per UoS were more than budgeted, the labor efficiency variance is unfavorable, as shown in Table 5.7.

Volume Variance

Volume variance measures the impact of volume on the department's financial performance. It measures a change in labor expense that can be attributed to a volume increase requiring more labor or a decrease requiring less labor.

BOX 5.2

CALCULATING LABOR VOLUME VARIANCE

Budgeted labor to produce actual UoS – Budgeted labor hours to produce budgeted UoS × Budgeted labor rate
Actual labor cost – Budgeted labor cost × Total labor hours

Applying the formula provided in Box 5.2 and using the data provided in Exhibit 5.7, the labor efficiency rate variance for the department is calculated as follows:

4,893 hours	Budgeted labor hours to produce actual UoS
− 4,742 hours	Budgeted labor hours to produce budgeted UoS
151	Labor volume variance

× $37.83	Budgeted labor rate
$5,712	Volume variance (Unfavorable)

Since the effect on labor hours was less than budgeted, the labor expense volume variance is unfavorable, as shown in Table 5.8.

Combined, the three types of variances equal the total labor expense variance, shown in Table 5.9. The casual observer may attribute the unfavorable labor expense variance to the increased surgical volume. However, upon further analysis by variance type, it is noteworthy that only 13% of the variance is due to increased volume. More than 50% of the variance is attributed to salary rates, such as overtime and contract labor. More than one third of the variance is due to productivity, such as staffing to the demand or inefficient workflows. Techniques to address both of these common causes of labor expense variance are discussed in Chapter 6.

TABLE 5.8 **Labor Expense Volume Variance Description**

VOLUME VARIANCE	
Favorable	Effect on labor hours was less than budgeted
Unfavorable	Effect on labor hours was more than budgeted

TABLE 5.9 **Labor Expense Variance**

TYPE	VARIANCE AMOUNT	PERCENT OF TOTAL VARIANCE
Rate	$23,377	52.5%
Efficiency	$15,435	34.7%
Volume	$5,712	12.8%
Total	$44,524	100.0%

STEP 3B. Determining Non-Labor Expense Variance (Figure 5.6)

The second largest category of operating expense over which healthcare leaders can directly influence or exert control is non-labor expense, such as supplies and purchased services. Similar to labor expense there are the three same categories for non-labor expense variance. Non-labor price or rate variance measures the impact of supply price on the department's performance.

The Department of Surgical Services has a total supply expense variance of $52,306 for the month, shown in Exhibit 5.9.

EXHIBIT 5.9

SUPPLY EXPENSE DETAIL FOR REGIONAL HEALTH SYSTEM'S DEPARTMENT OF SURGICAL SERVICES

SEPTEMBER FY 20X2

Medical Supplies	Actual	Budget	Variance	% Variance	
Medical supply cost	$ 223,896	$ 179,394	$ (44,502)	−24.8%	U
Units of supply	2,231	2,000	(231)	−11.6%	U

UoS	Actual	Budget	Variance	% Variance	
Procedures (adjusted)	699	670	29	4.3%	F
Supply cost per unit	$ 100.36	$ 89.70	$ (10.66)	−11.9%	U
Supplies per UoS	3.19	2.99	(0.2)	−6.9%	U

1. Price (or Rate) Variance		
Actual supply cost per unit	$ 100.36	U
Budgeted supply cost per unit	$ 89.70	U
Rate variance	$ (10.66)	
Actual units of supply used	2,231	
	$ (23,782)	U
2. Efficiency Variance		
Actual supplies to produce actual UoS	2,231	
Budgeted supplies to produce actual UoS	2,000	U
Supply usage variance	231	
Budgeted supply cost per unit	$ 89.70	
	$ 20,720	U
3. Volume Variance		
Budgeted supplies to produce actual UoS	2,087	
Budgeted supplies to produce budgeted UoS	2,000	U
Supply volume variance	87	U
Budgeted supply cost per unit	$ 89.70	
	$ 7,804	U
Total non-labor (supply) expense variance	$ 52,306	U

F, favorable variance; U, unfavorable variance; UoS, units of service.

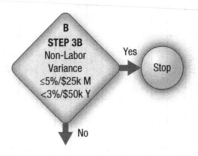

FIGURE 5.6 Step 3B: Determining non-labor expense variance.
M, month; Y, year.

Applying the formula provided in Box 5.3 and using the data provided in Table 5.10, the supply rate variance for the department is calculated as follows:

$100.36	Actual supply cost per hour
− $89.70	Budgeted supply cost per hour
(10.66)	Supply rate variance (actual vs. budgeted supply cost)
× 2,231	Actual units of supply used
$23,782	Rate variance (Unfavorable)

Since the supply price per unit was more than budgeted, the supply expense rate variance is unfavorable, as shown in Table 5.10.

Efficiency variance measures the effect of supply usage on the department's financial performance. This measure is used to assess how effectively the department is staffing to meet the volume demands of the department.

BOX 5.3

CALCULATING SUPPLY RATE VARIANCE

Actual supply cost per unit − Budgeted supply cost per unit
    × Actual units of supply used
Actual labor cost − Budgeted labor cost × Total labor hours

TABLE 5.10 **Supply Rate Variance Description**

RATE VARIANCE	
Favorable	Supply price per unit was less than budgeted
Unfavorable	Supply price per unit was more than budgeted

Applying the formula provided in Box 5.4 and using the data provided in Exhibit 5.9 the supply rate variance for the department is calculated as follows:

BOX 5.4

CALCULATING SUPPLY EFFICIENCY VARIANCE

Actual supplies to produce actual UoS – Budgeted supplies to produce actual
   UoS × Budgeted supply cost per unit
Actual labor cost – Budgeted labor cost × Total labor hours

2,231 units	Actual supplies to produce actual UoS	⎰ Budgeted supplies per UoS (2.99) × Procedures (699)
– 2,000 units	Budgeted supplies to produce actual UoS	
231	Supply usage variance	
× $89.70	Budgeted supply cost per unit	
$20,720	Efficiency variance (Unfavorable)	

Since the supplies per UoS were more than budgeted the supply expense efficiency variance is unfavorable, as shown in Table 5.11.

Volume variance measures the effect of volume on the department's financial performance; that is, a change in supply expense that can be attributed to a volume increase requiring more supplies or services or a decrease requiring less supplies and services.

TABLE 5.11 **Supply Efficiency Variance Description**

EFFICIENCY VARIANCE	
Favorable	Supplies per UoS were less than budgeted
Unfavorable	Supplies per UoS were more than budgeted

BOX 5.5

CALCULATING SUPPLY VOLUME VARIANCE

Budgeted supplies to produce actual UoS – Budgeted supplies to produce
   budgeted UoS × Budgeted supply cost per unit
Actual labor cost – Budgeted labor cost × Total labor hours

Applying the formula provided in Box 5.5 and using the data provided in Exhibit 5.9, the supply volume variance for the department is calculated as follows:

2,087 units	Budgeted supplies to produce actual UoS
− 2,000 units	Budgeted supplies to produce budgeted UoS
87	Supply volume variance
× $89.70	Budgeted supply cost per unit
$7,804	Volume variance (Unfavorable)

Since the effect on supplies was less than budgeted the supply expense volume variance is unfavorable, as shown in Table 5.12.

Combined, the three types variances equal the total supply expense variance, shown in Table 5.13. Techniques to address common causes of non-labor expense variance are discussed in Chapter 7.

TABLE 5.12 **Supply Volume Variance Description**

VOLUME VARIANCE	
Favorable	Effect on supplies was less than budgeted
Unfavorable	Effect on supplies was more than budgeted

TABLE 5.13 **Supply Expense Variance**

TYPE	VARIANCE AMOUNT	PERCENT OF TOTAL VARIANCE
Rate	$23,782	45.5%
Efficiency	$20,720	39.6%
Volume	$7,804	14.9%
Total	$52,306	100.0%

STEP 4. Determining Root Cause of Variance

After determining the variance source, such as labor or non-labor, and the category (rate, productivity, or volume), the next step is to collect and assess the necessary data to determine the root cause of any variance exceeding the financial pathway threshold (Figure 5.7). This requires additional information beyond what is provided in the P&L statement. Effective analysis typically requires the subject matter expertise of a data analyst as well as functional expertise within the specific variance area, such as human resources or finance for labor expense variance and supply chain or materials management staff

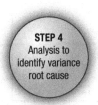

FIGURE 5.7 Step 4: Determining root cause of variance.

for non-labor variance. Both should be able to provide, validate, and interpret source data, such as timecards, overtime reports, and invoices.

STEP 5. Corrective Action Plan

Action planning is the final and most important step of the financial pathway process. Once the cause of the variance is identified the next to last step is developing and implementing a **corrective action plan**, as shown in Figure 5.8. The purpose of any action plan is to identify all of the required tasks to achieve the desired objectives to reduce or eliminate the variances identified in the previous steps. An effective action plan includes a projected completion date and assignment of the individual who will be primarily accountable for completing each task. The SMART objective format is a useful approach to help leaders define what they are trying to accomplish. Every sub-goal and objective supporting the larger strategic goal should be SMART: *s*pecific, *m*easurable, *a*chievable, *r*elevant, and *t*ime-oriented. The action plan example for the department is provided in Exhibit 5.10 (see also Table 5.14). An Action Plan template used in Exhibit 5.10 with guidelines for completing is available on Springer Connect (visit connect.springerpub.com/content/book/978-0-8261-4464-5/chapter/ch05 and access the show chapter supplementary dropdown at the beginning of the chapter).

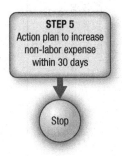

FIGURE 5.8 Step 5: Determining and implementing the corrective action plan.

EXHIBIT 5.10

STRATEGIC GOAL: REDUCE UNNECESSARY OPERATING EXPENSE BY 15% BY THE END OF THE FISCAL YEAR TO ACHIEVE ANNUAL BUDGET TARGET

GOAL	ACTIONS	TIMELINE AND STATUS		RESPONSIBLE	FINANCIAL IMPACT
Reduce overtime labor expense $23,363 by the end of the 4th quarter	a. Identify opportunities to reduce avoidable overtime expense	Oct. 10	Complete	Nancy W.	$12,316
	b. Review staffing levels and schedule to identify and eliminate avoidable overtime	Oct. 15		Nancy W.	N/A
	c. Implement employee accountability process for any overtime variance	Oct. 18		Peter M.	$7,104
	d. Review time cards daily of employees who consistently exceed scheduled shift hours	Oct. 20		Donna K.	$3,943
	e. Counsel employees who exceed scheduled shift hours	Oct. 25		Nancy W.	N/A

TABLE 5.14 **Steps for Developing the Corrective Action Plan**

Step 1	Identify strategic goal
Step 2	Identify sub-goals
Step 3	Identify supporting actions (tasks)
Step 4	Determine timeline for completion
Step 5	Identify individual responsible for completing each task
Step 6	Calculate financial impact

SUMMARY

Healthcare leaders responsible and accountable for the financial and operations performance of a business enterprise are in an environment of increasing pressure on operating margins. Accordingly, leaders must adopt a deliberate and systematic approach to achieve specific financial targets communicated in the budget. Using the financial pathway as a framework to identify, prioritize, manage, and reduce unfavorable variances will enable leaders' making effective decisions that achieve the strategic goals of the organization and improve financial performance. Identifying and prioritizing financial variances to better tailor action planning efforts that address the specific root causes eliminates time-consuming and costly guesswork and trial and error.

CALLS TO ACTION

Leaders should:

- Use the financial pathway to identify and prioritize financial variances.
- Adopt the MOR and action plan to provide a framework for promoting accountability to improve financial and operations performance.
- Continuously measure, monitor, and proactively manage departments through the action planning process

Reference

1. Perry J, Mobley F, Brubaker M. Most doctors have little or no management training, and that's a problem. *Harvard Business Review*. December 15, 2017.

PART IV

MANAGING

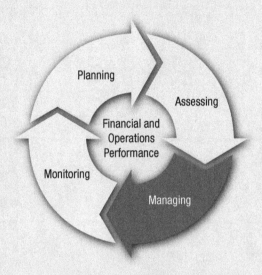

INTRODUCTION TO MANAGING

Managing involves the range of actions taken by healthcare leaders to guide and drive performance improvement opportunities identified during the Assessing Phase of the Effective Financial and Operations Management Cycle. Managing financial performance requires understanding the key drivers and then developing and decisively implementing a corrective action plan. Managing increasingly scarce resources to improve the healthcare provider organization's financial and operations performance involves two primary actions: reducing unnecessary operating expense and growing incremental revenue.

CHAPTER 6

MANAGING LABOR PRODUCTIVITY AND EXPENSE

LEARNING OBJECTIVES

- Use effective tactics to manage labor productivity and expense.
- Apply a span of control analysis to flatten unproductive and costly management layers.
- Design an open position review process to proactively evaluate opportunities to reduce labor expense.

TOOLS AND TECHNIQUES

- Labor productivity analysis
- Managing labor productivity and expense
- Staffing to demand
- Open position review
- Span of control analysis
- Measuring financial impact of improving labor productivity and expense

KEY TERMS AND CONCEPTS

Labor productivity

Labor rate

Skill mix

Exempt

Non-exempt

Full-time equivalent (FTE)

Paid hours

Productive hours

Non-productive hours

Labor ratio

INTRODUCTION

The healthcare industry is labor intensive requiring a professional, highly-skilled, and expensive workforce. Effectively managing labor productivity is a critical leadership skill with the goal of getting the right number and mix of staff at the right time and place to provide the highest quality and most accessible service possible (Box 6.1). **Labor productivity** is the effective and efficient use of human resources or the staff for which leaders are accountable to accomplish their organization's mission. Proactively managing labor productivity has the most significant and favorable impact on the business enterprise's financial performance. Staffing is the most critical function over which leaders have control and accountability; however it is often misunderstood and mismanaged causing poor quality, inefficiency, and strained financial performance. There are many common challenges to effective labor productivity.

BOX 6.1

GOALS OF MANAGING LABOR PRODUCTIVITY

- Right amount of staff
- Right skill mix
- Right time
- Right place

CHALLENGES TO MANAGING LABOR PRODUCTIVITY

The demand for healthcare services can be unpredictable and vary widely due to seasonality. Demand fluctuations are exacerbated by multiple, often inefficient processes and inputs, including patient needs, provider and staff availability, and access to the necessary equipment, services, and supplies. Also, complex, onerous, and sub-optimal workflows can impact effective labor productivity, further challenging leaders' ability to use labor resources efficiently.

Variation in volume demand can cause inefficient and costly overstaffing or understaffing. Among the common challenges leaders face managing labor productivity are wasted staff time handing-off care from one provider to another and bottlenecks from waiting for test results or for care to be delivered. There are also challenges in coordinating the multitude of activities across various often siloed departments and functions, both care-related and non-care related, many of which do not lend any value to the intended outcome.

The biggest challenge leaders face is managing staffing levels to meet varying demands.

LEADERS' ROLE IN MANAGING LABOR PRODUCTIVITY

Leaders have influence in recruiting the right staff, developing them, and setting and adjusting staffing levels and skill mix to avoid or reduce unnecessary labor expense (Box 6.2).

BOX 6.2

LEADER RESPONSIBILITIES FOR MANAGING LABOR PRODUCTIVITY
1. Hiring and on-boarding
2. Training and education
3. Labor rate
4. Staffing levels
5. Skill mix
6. Workflow

There are many factors that impact labor productivity over which leaders have control or influence. First is the recruitment and on-boarding process for new employees to ensure the right fit for the specific needs of each job. Hiring manager leaders are responsible for making sure the job description and desired qualifications closely match the incumbent hired. Next leaders must invest in the continuous professional development of all staff through value-added orientation, training, and education.

The **labor rate** includes salary or wages and all benefits paid to staff. The salary or hourly rate paid to employees is largely determined by fair market value and the supply and demand for the specific skill set. While human resources is responsible for establishing competitive pay rates for the various job classifications, leaders can control labor expense by managing staffing levels. Staffing is the direct responsibility of leaders and should be based on deliberate and quantitative criteria, such as an acuity-adjusted staffing grid or matrix with established minimum "core-level" staffing to ensure patient safety. Staffing should be continuously adjusted according to patient volume and acuity.

EXHIBIT 6.1

SKILL MIX FINANCIAL IMPACT EXAMPLE (NURSING MODELS)

NURSING MODEL	SKILL LEVEL	FULL-TIME EQUIVALENTS	HOURLY RATE	TOTAL HOURS	ANNUAL EXPENSE
1. All RN	RN	30	$ 35.00	62,400	$ 2,184,000
2. RN-LVN mix	RN	9	$ 20.00	18,720	$ 374,400
	LVN	21	$ 35.00	43,680	$ 1,528,800
					$ 1,903,200
		Annual labor expense savings			$ 280,800

Another leadership consideration is skill mix. **Skill mix** is having the right employee for the right task. Leaders should balance their staffing skill mix so that all employees are working at the "top of their license." Achieving this balance is challenging and has significant financial implications. For example, assume a licensed vocational nurse (LVN) earns $20 an hour to administer basic nursing care such as checking vital signs, changing bandages, and bathing patients. A registered nurse (RN) provides a more advanced level of care and makes $35 per hour. The potential financial impact of using an RN–LVN nursing skill mix model versus an "all RN" model is illustrated in Exhibit 6.1.

Assuming 30% of an RN's total duties could be accomplished by an LVN and factoring the amount of an RN's time required to supervise the work of an LVN, the RN–LVN model is a great example of managing staff skill mix to improve labor productivity. The projected annual savings in this example is $280,800 determined by calculating the difference between the cost of the RN model and the RN–LVN model. Another potential benefit is the likely positive impact on improving nursing morale and decreasing involuntary turnover.

The same logic and potential for significant savings applies to other interdisciplinary collaborative support models, including physicians and physician assistants, physical therapists and physician therapy assistants, and pharmacists and pharmacy technicians. Another staffing consideration is the mix of full-time, part-time, and per diem (as needed) employees. Having a balance of each category allows flexibility to increase or decrease staffing to match demand. Using a mix of full- and part-time or per diem employees allows the ability to flex down during slow periods without incurring the labor expense of having more full-time staff than necessary. A reasonable mix is 70% full-time staff and 30% part-time and per diem employees.

MEASURING AND EVALUATING LABOR PRODUCTIVITY

Before being able to adequately measure labor productivity, leaders must first distinguish between exempt and non-exempt employees. **Exempt** employees typically receive a fixed salary regardless of the number of hours they work per week, usually have some managerial responsibilities, and are not entitled to overtime pay. Alternatively, **non-exempt** employees are compensated on an hourly basis and paid overtime usually for working more than 40 hours per week. The focus of most labor management efforts are on non-exempt employees since their scheduling and associated compensation are typically dependent upon patient volume.

The standard unit of labor measurement is the **full-time equivalent** or FTE. FTEs convert part-time employees into full-time employees. For example, two part-time employees working half-time each would equal one FTE. Typically an FTE is comprised of 2,080 total paid hours where the employee works an average of 40 hours per week over the year. An example of an exempt employee is one FTE medical technologist supervisor who is paid a fixed annual salary of $62,500 and expected to work an average of 45 to 50 hours each week without receiving any overtime.

Total **paid hours** can be further broken down into productive and non-productive hours. **Productive hours** include all employee work activities including breaks and lunch. **Non-productive hours** are all of the non-work activities such as paid time off (PTO) or vacation, sick time, bereavement, orientation, education, and training. Table 6.1 provides an example of how an FTE is calculated.

The ratio of productive to non-productive hours is dependent upon how generous the healthcare provider organization's benefits are and typically vary according to how long the employee has been with the organization. The accrual of PTO typically increases with an employee's years of service as a retention incentive. To illustrate how to calculate a non-exempt FTE, one FTE medical technologist is hired at the base rate of $25.00 per hour. The employee is scheduled to work 8 hours a day 5 days per week. To determine the employee's total annual wages the number of hours is multiplied by the hourly rate. The medical technologist is paid an annual gross amount of $52,000, excluding taxes and benefits paid by the organization. The organization offers new employees

TABLE 6.1 **Calculating Full-Time Equivalent (Paid and Productive Hours)**

TIME UNIT	TOTAL PAID HOURS	CALCULATION
Day	8	8 hours per day
Week	40	5 days x 8 hours
Year	2,080	40 hours per week x 52 weeks per year

TABLE 6.2 **Full-Time Equivalent Calculation Example**

ACTIVITY	TYPE OF HOURS	NUMBER OF PAID HOURS PER YEAR	NUMBER OF PAID 8-HOUR DAYS PER YEAR
Total paid hours and days		2,080 hours	260 days
Scheduled work	Productive	1,872 hours	234 days
Vacation	Non-productive	80 hours	10 days
Holidays	Non-productive	56 hours	7 days
Sick and bereavement leave	Non-productive	40 hours	5 days
Orientation, education, and training	Non-productive	32 hours	4 days

2 weeks (10 days) of paid vacation per year. In addition, the organization offers 7 paid federal holidays and 5 days of combined sick and bereavement leave. New hire orientation or education and training are another 4 days per year. The organization categorizes employee time as shown in Table 6.2.

Of the total 2,080 hours the employee is paid each year the amount of schedulable work time is 1,872 hours or 234 days. Another 26 days are paid to the employee but are non-productive. The remaining 104 are unpaid days or days off, usually the weekend or other 2 days the employee is not scheduled to work. The ratio of productive to non-productive time is 90:10 as shown in Figure 6.1. Measuring labor productivity involves determining the specific amount of staff time required to provide services. Greater labor efficiency lends to higher productivity, capacity, and financial performance. Because labor is the key input in the provision of healthcare services, labor productivity is the primary focus of the efficiency measurement.

LABOR PRODUCTIVITY ANALYSIS

The most commonly used labor performance measurement indicators involve some volume statistic per productive hour or actual worked hour such as the

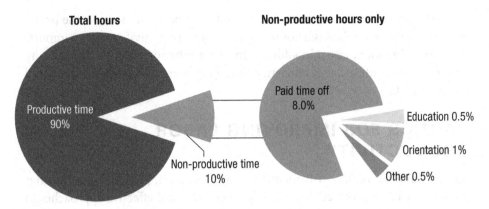

FIGURE 6.1 Productive and non-productive hours.

number of productive hours to produce an inpatient discharge, outpatient clinic visit, surgical procedure, or diagnostic test. National comparative labor benchmarks, such as ActionOI, can be useful if the comparative peer group reflects the specific characteristics of the healthcare provider organization. Otherwise such benchmarks are relatively meaningless since each organization has different requirements and sometimes unique challenges that prevent useful comparisons. Internal benchmarks that are aligned with the healthcare provider organization's budget targets and compared or trended over time are the most useful and actionable. Benchmarking is discussed further in Chapter 10.

The industry standard labor efficiency measure is the **labor ratio** shown in Box 6.3. A rule-of-thumb best practice for healthcare provider organizations is a labor ratio of 40% or less. Poorer performers have a ratio of 60% or higher.

BOX 6.3

CALCULATING LABOR RATIO

$$\text{Labor ratio} = \frac{\text{Total labor cost}}{\text{Total revenue}}$$

There are other measures of labor productivity and efficiency that either use FTEs to measure the amount of labor used or some resource-denominated measure, such as paid hours per inpatient discharge and the number of FTEs per occupied bed. These measures assess the productivity of labor devoted to inpatient services as a function of the number of patients. Because the provision of inpatient services is labor intensive, labor productivity plays an important role in inpatient costs. In addition to the number of patients, the intensity of services also affects labor efficiency. These ratios are discussed in more detail in Chapter 4.

TACTICS FOR IMPROVING LABOR PRODUCTIVITY

Leaders should continuously identify, prioritize, and implement opportunities to improve labor productivity. Identifying creative and effective approaches to reduce unnecessary operating expense without compromising quality, safety, and access is a common challenge for many leaders. A comprehensive list of proven effective approaches used in top-performing healthcare provider organizations is provided in Appendix E. The top five most impactful tactics for improving labor productivity listed in Box 6.4 include controlling avoidable overtime, assessing non-productive paid time such as meetings, staffing to demand, evaluating open positions, and revising the organization chart using a span of control analysis.

BOX 6.4

KEY DRIVERS FOR IMPROVING LABOR PRODUCTIVITY
1. Eliminate unnecessary overtime
2. Assess opportunities to reduce orientation, education, training, and meetings
3. Staff to demand
4. Evaluate open positions
5. Re-engineer organization chart

Eliminate Overtime

Overtime (OT) is often a necessary evil although an inefficient and expensive use of scarce resources. OT is typically paid at 1-1/2 or even 2 times the normal hourly rate. Healthcare provider organizations are often challenged with accurately measuring, reporting, and managing overtime payment. The causes of high OT expense greater than 3% of the total labor expense for the business enterprise should be closely examined to understand the specific causes. The common and avoidable reasons for high OT include excessive open positions, lack of discipline in employee clocking-in and out, and allowing employees to schedule themselves for overtime shifts on a "first-come-first-served" basis. All of these require tight management controls to limit overtime expense.

Reduce Orientation, Education, Training, and Meetings

The judicious use of training, orientation, education, and meetings is a significant opportunity to improve labor productivity. Healthcare provider organizations are increasingly moving training into virtual classrooms that employees can complete at their own pace and at significantly less expense. Executives spend nearly 23 hours a week in meetings, not including unscheduled impromptu meetings. What's more, 71% believed the meetings were unproductive.[1] A good litmus test to apply for holding a meeting is if the information can be disseminated using another medium, such as an electronic newsletter or online bulletin board. Meetings should only be held when there is a need for active engagement of key stakeholders to make or recommend a decision. Even so, every meeting should have a written agenda with its purpose and goals sent to invitees at least 1 week in advance, include the right people to make or recommend decisions, start and end on time, and be followed-up shortly afterward with concise documentation of the discussion, key decisions made or recommended, and next steps.

Staffing to Demand

The common resource-denominated approach to staffing can be a useful productivity measure. However, it is largely focused on an hours per unit of service volume statistic discussed in Chapter 4. Staffing is therefore scheduled based on traditional shifts, such as those shown in Table 6.3.

Unfortunately, the traditional staffing approach largely ignores the ability to respond to fluctuating demand. Volume levels can have significant and often unpredictable swings, the impact of which creates waste and adds unnecessary labor expense. Traditional staffing models focus largely on the total cost of labor versus only productive hours. The end result is either over-staffing or under-staffing causing inefficient use of costly resources or an unsafe

TABLE 6.3 Traditional Staffing

SHIFT	START	END
Day	7 am	3 pm
Evening	3 pm	11 pm
Night	11 pm	7 am

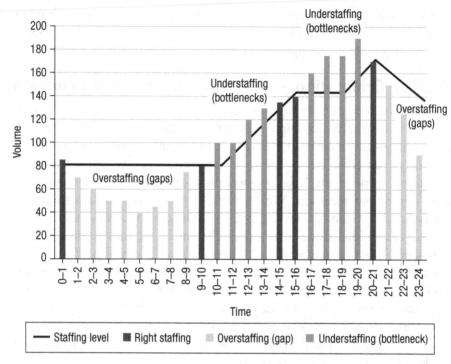

FIGURE 6.2 Staffing challenges due to volume demand fluctuation.

environment that could cause harm to patients. The resulting waiting, delays, and bottlenecks are also a significant dissatisfier for staff.

Figure 6.2 shows a typical hour-by-hour variation in patient volume compared to traditional staffing levels. Note the understaffing (bottlenecks) and overstaffing (gaps) that occur, potentially adversely impacting quality and service. Armed with this type of information leaders can adjust their staffing grids and schedules to better reflect demand. Leaders can also improve labor productivity, quality, and safety by better organizing the work more efficiently through "shaping demand." Shaping or smoothing demand is accomplished through several simple techniques, including performing schedulable work during predictable slow periods, such as patient callbacks, inventory, paperwork and delaying non-critical tasks to slower times of the day, week, or month.

An alternative to traditional shift staffing is varying or "flexing" staff according to volume demands. As staff are reallocated or flexed to overburdened times of the day, healthcare provider organizations will find that labor productivity can be dramatically improved with a significant impact on financial performance from reducing labor expense. Following the Lean-Six Sigma engineering Failure Modes Effects Analysis (FMEA) concept popularized by The Joint Commission, leaders can conduct three critical actions to better align their staffing with demand, presented in Box 6.5. The ultimate impact of these three actions enables leaders' focus to shift from a traditional resource-denominated approach to a more manageable process-denominated approach.

BOX 6.5

STEPS FOR STAFFING TO DEMAND
1. Identify historical staffing bottlenecks and gaps on an hour-by-hour basis.
2. Redesign staffing plans around patient demand rather than traditional shift scheduling.
3. Make and monitor staffing changes as needed.

Staffing to demand by flexing staff can also be applied in all areas of the healthcare provider organization, including outpatient clinics and surgery. The key to success in flexing staff is setting the expectation upfront, ideally during the hiring process to avoid employees staying clocked-in to get their 40 hours per week even though their work is done. A best practice approach is to sign "guarantee" letters for employees in areas where there are frequent gaps and bottlenecks causing slack time when they could be flexed off and bottlenecks when they might incur overtime. The hospital operating room is a common example where expensive resources are typically only 50% utilized. The expectation set with employees is there will be times when their workload is completed prior to their schedule shift ending, assuming there isn't a valid need in another area, in which case they can either go home or use PTO. Also, there will be occasions when they will be asked to stay late and be eligible for overtime pay. Regardless, the guarantee letter stipulates the organization will pay their full FTE wages for the year if there is any shortfall. This eliminates employees' concern of not getting enough hours to pay their bills and avoids their getting paid not to work or potentially gaming the system.

Open Position Review

A number of opportunities present when a position becomes vacant for whatever reason. Top-performing healthcare provider organizations have a disciplined process for reviewing open or vacant positions involving a meeting between the hiring manager leader and the direct report executive as part of an "open" or "vacant position committee." The open position committee is typically comprised of senior executive leaders such as the chief financial officer, chief nursing officer, and the chief operating officer. The committee reviews all requests to fill open positions at least monthly. It is responsible for ensuring that the position is necessary and there are no other creative ways to fill or merge the position by asking the five questions listed in Box 6.6. This process promotes active and effective labor productivity management and reduces unnecessary waste and expense.

BOX 6.6

OPEN POSITION QUESTION CHECKLIST
1. Can the position be eliminated?
2. Can the position be made part-time or PRN?
3. Can the functions of the position be assigned to another person?
4. Can the functions of the position be batched for completion?
5. Can the functions of the position be assigned to a high-performer ("A" leader) with growth capacity?

Span of Control Analysis

Many healthcare provider organizations are top heavy in their management ranks. Management positions are often created to provide professional growth through internal promotion opportunities to retain good staff without regard for the impact on organizational decision-making efficiency. Too many managerial layers can create wasteful meetings and non-value added work. "Flattening" the management structure through a span of control analysis can improve decision-making efficiency and reduce unnecessary labor expense. The steps for conducting the span of control analysis are listed in Box 6.7.

The first step in the span of control analysis is to replicate the current organization chart of the business enterprise or of the larger organization on a white board or flip chart with sticky notes with the name and position of each leader. Next, each leadership position from vice president to manager should be reviewed and scrutinized with the executive leader to whom they report. "De-coupling" the organization chart allows leaders to understand the many, sometimes hidden, layers of management that exist. During the review process the same questions are asked about each leadership position as for the open position review in Box 6.6.

The next step is for each position to be objectively and confidentially assigned an "A," "B," or "C." "A" leaders are the top-performers who have the capability and the capacity to increase their level of responsibility, possibly with some consideration for additional compensation. "B" leaders are recognized solid performers in the organization who can be groomed with additional mentoring and training to become an "A" leader. "B" leaders may be able to assume

> **BOX 6.7**
>
> **STEPS FOR CONDUCTING A SPAN OF CONTROL ANALYSIS**
> 1. Replicate the organizational chart on a white board.
> 2. Label each position with the name and title of each position's manager and above (1 up, 2 down).
> 3. Identify each leader as "A," "B," or "C."
> 4. Re-engineer (flatten) the organizational chart based on opportunities to promote "A" and "B" leaders and outplace "C" leaders.

additional responsibility. "C" leaders may not be in the right role or possibly the right organization and should be considered for outplacement.

According to Jim Collins, great leaders first get the right people on the bus and the wrong people off the bus.[2] Increasing leaders' span of control ideally to four to six direct reports provides an opportunity to flatten the organizational hierarchy while providing top-performing "A" leaders with professional development and growth opportunities. Outplacing non-performing "C" leaders sets and communicates clear performance expectations and the consequences for failing to meet them. Examples of the organizational chart before and after the span of control analysis are presented in Figures 6.3 and 6.4, respectively. The flattened organizational structure creates increased decision-making efficiency and eliminates unnecessary expense.

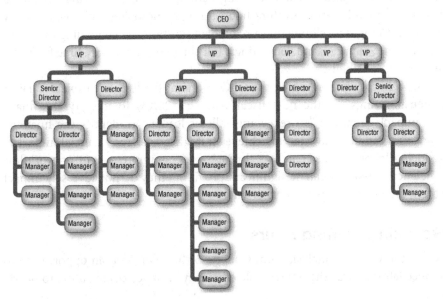

FIGURE 6.3 Organizational chart before span of control analysis.

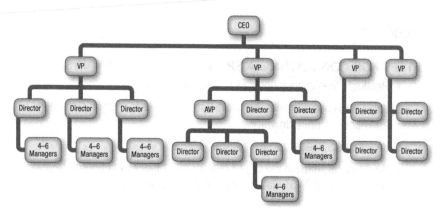

FIGURE 6.4 Organizational chart after span of control analysis.

REGIONAL HEALTH SYSTEM CASE EXAMPLE: REDUCING LABOR EXPENSE

Under continued pressure to reduce unnecessary operating expense and considering the insight from completing the financial condition analysis addressed in Chapter 4, the Director of Surgical Services for Regional Health System (RHS) assessed quickly implementable opportunities to improve labor productivity and reduce expense. Among the options she identified that will have the greatest impact within the next quarter include reducing staffing hours by improving scheduling to match demand, cutting overtime hours through improving workflow efficiency and monitoring staff, eliminating a redundant position and combining the duties with another manager, and converting a full-time position to part-time for better staffing mix flexibility.

The Director was asked by the CFO to quantify all of her projected labor expense savings for the next fiscal year (FY 20X3) to identify the financial impact. Financial "scorekeeping" allows leaders to identify the financial gains that can be reinvested to achieve strategic goals. The financial impact of reducing labor expense, such as through process improvement or workflow efficiency initiatives, can be significant providing they do not adversely impact safety, quality, or the patient experience.

Reducing Staffing Hours

Recall the variance analysis from Chapter 5 that identified an opportunity to reduce labor hours. The unfavorable efficiency variance contributing to nearly

35% of the total variance for September 20X2 was 559 paid hours shown in Exhibit 6.2.

Implementing scheduling changes to better match staffing levels with the surgical volume, the Director plans to reduce the average staff time per adjusted case by 7.5% equaling $69,841 in annual labor expense savings. The methodology shown in Exhibit 6.3 calculates the change impact and anticipated annualized savings for the next fiscal year from decreasing the paid hours per adjusted case. Calculating the annual impact from reducing the required labor hours by 0.57 results in a $296 savings per adjusted case and $69,841 savings for the next fiscal year (FY 20X3).

EXHIBIT 6.2

MONTHLY LABOR EXPENSE DETAIL FOR REGIONAL HEALTH SYSTEM'S DEPARTMENT OF SURGICAL SERVICES

SEPTEMBER FY 20X2				
Labor Expense	Actual	Budget	Variance	% Variance
Director	$8,444	$8,444	$ -	0.0%
RN	$172,190	$131,845	$ (40,345)	−30.6%
LVN	$31,238	$27,800	$ (3,438)	−12.4%
Aide	$8,712	$7,993	$ (719)	−9.0%
Clerical	$3,312	$3,312	$ -	0.0%
Total Labor Expense	$223,896	$179,394	$ (44,502)	−24.8%
Labor Hours				
Director	160	160	0	0.0%
RN	3,280	2,848	(432)	−15.2%
LVN	1,144	910	(234)	−25.7%
Aide	477	584	107	18.3%
Clerical	240	240	0	0.0%
Total Labor Hours	5,301	4,742	(559)	−11.8%
Units of Service (UoS)				
Procedures (adjusted)	699	670	29	4.3%
Labor cost per hour	$42.24	$37.83	$ (4.41)	−11.7%
Labor hours per UoS	7.58	7.00	(0.58)	−8.3%

EXHIBIT 6.3

PROJECTED ANNUAL LABOR EXPENSE SAVINGS FROM REDUCING STAFFING HOURS

SEPTEMBER FY 20X2	
Units of service (adjusted procedures)	699
Total labor hours	5,301
Labor hours per adjusted case	7.58
Labor cost per hour	$42.24
Labor cost per adjusted case	$320
Total labor expense	$223,914
Labor hour reduction (per case)	**7.5%**
Revised total labor hours	4,903
Revised labor hours per adjusted case	7.01
Labor cost per hour	$42.24
Revised labor cost per adjusted case	$296
Revised total labor expense	$ 207,121
Cost savings	**$ 16,794**

Reducing Overtime (OT) Hours

The labor rate variance identified from the Director's analysis for September FY 20X2 was $23,377, contributing to more than half of the total labor expense variance for the month. Labor expense includes paid wages and overtime (OT) for non-exempt or hourly employees. The total number of OT hours was 666 hours: 432 for RNs and 234 for LVNs in September 20X2, reflecting 1 hour of OT for every adjusted case. The contributing RN overtime was 77% of the total amount and 23% for LVNs.

By streamlining critical workflow processes and monitoring employee clocking-in and out according to the newly published policy and procedures, the Director plans to reduce total OT hours by 20% for both types of nurses totaling $34,180 in annual labor expense savings. She assumes that all shifts are fully staffed and the reduction of OT eliminates the additional hour that created the premium pay. Recall that employee OT is paid 50% more for the same productivity and therefore contributes to very inefficient use of staffing as shown in Table 6.4.

TABLE 6.4 **Calculating the Overtime Rate for Employees**

EMPLOYEE TYPE	BASE RATE PER HOUR	OVERTIME EXPENSE PER HOUR	TOTAL OVERTIME RATE PER HOUR
RN	$43.05	$21.53	$64.58
LVN	$22.39	$11.20	$33.59

With the OT rate of 1 hour per adjusted case, the projected annual financial impact of reducing OT hours is calculated by determining the expected number of RN and LVN OT hours using the provided percent for each. Without the Director's plan to reduce OT expense, the expected number of OT hours in FY 20X3 would be 2,907 hours based on the budgeted 2,907 adjusted case volume. The cost of the unmanaged OT is calculated by multiplying the OT rate per hour by the number of OT hours for each equaling $144,530 for RNs and $26,368 for LVNs. Reducing the total projected $170,898 OT expense by 20% would equal $34,180 in annual labor expense savings.

Eliminating a Position

Based on the opportunity to combine two positions by assigning additional responsibilities to an "A" employee identified from the span of control analysis previously presented, the Director plans to eliminate one FTE position saving $35,170 in the first year and $49,560 in the following years. When calculating the financial impact of eliminating a position that is currently filled there are four components to consider: salary or wages, benefits, any severance paid, and accrued PTO that needs to be paid. The manager position being eliminated has an annual salary of $49,560 that includes $42,000 base plus 18% benefits. The employee occupying the position will receive a 3-month severance equaling $12,390 plus an additional $2,000 for accrued paid time off. The annualized first year savings is calculated by subtracting the severance and PTO from the total salary and benefits, which is $35,170.

Converting a Position From Full-Time to Part-Time

In the last opportunity to reduce labor expense the Director identified a full-time position that can be converted to part-time to provide more scheduling flexibility, saving an additional $20,617 per year. The current 1.0 FTE position will be changed to a 0.70 FTE, or from 40 to 28 hours per week. The hourly rate for this position is $28 plus 18% benefits equaling $68,723 annually. The position is still eligible for benefits. The 0.30 FTE reduction is a $20,617 labor expense savings.

TABLE 6.5 **Planned Labor Expense Initiatives and Projected Financial Impact**

LABOR EXPENSE REDUCTION INITIATIVE	FINANCIAL IMPACT
1. Implement schedule changes to better match staffing levels with the surgical volume demand reducing the average time per adjusted case by 7.5%.	$69,841
2. Streamline critical workflow processes and monitor employee clocking-in and out to reduce overtime by 20%.	$34,180
3. Eliminate manager position by combining two positions through assigning additional responsibility to an "A" employee identified from the span of control analysis.	$35,170
4. Convert a full-time position to part-time providing more scheduling flexibility to match volume demand.	$20,617
Total projected annual labor expense reduction	$159,808

The total projected annual cost savings opportunity for FY 20X3 resulting from the Director's initiatives is $159,808, summarized in Table 6.5. The labor expense savings are not achieved until the detailed corrective action plans are developed, implemented, and closely monitored as addressed in Chapter 5. Whenever expense reduction opportunities involve other departments and leaders, involving key stakeholders to get their buy-in and support is critical to success.

SUMMARY

Effectively managing labor productivity is a critical leadership skill with the goal of getting the right number and mix of staff at the right time and place to provide high quality, safe, and accessible care. Leaders accountable for the financial and operations performance of a business enterprise can apply proven effective tactics to improve labor productivity and reduce expense, including staffing to demand, conducting open position reviews, and doing a span of control analysis. All labor productivity improvement initiatives must be "scored" to estimate the planned financial impact. Once implemented through the corrective action plan, improvement initiatives must be closely monitored and managed to achieve the desired results.

CALLS TO ACTION

Leaders should:

- Recognize the significant impact improving labor productivity has on reducing operating expense and achieving financial performance goals.

■ Implement proven effective tactics for improving labor productivity, including an open position review committee and span of control analysis.

■ Monetize labor expense reduction initiatives to monitor the savings contribution to financial performance improvement and goals and the investment potential in quality and safety.

References

1. Perlow LA, Hadley CN, Eun E. (2017). Stop the meeting madness. *Harvard Business Review*, July-August.
2. Collins JC. *Good to Great: Why Some Companies Make the Leap...and Others Don't.* Harper Business; 2001.

CHAPTER 7

MANAGING NON-LABOR PRODUCTIVITY AND EXPENSE

Market-share pricing	Value analysis process (VAP)
Request for proposal (RFP)	Value analysis team (VAT)
Best and final offer (BAFO)	Insourcing
Demand matching	Outsourcing

INTRODUCTION

Healthcare provider organizations are experiencing rising supply and service costs contributing to an increasing share of their operating expense. The rapid proliferation of medical science and technology introducing costly new treatments and drugs is further driving up unreimbursable costs. **Non-labor productivity** is the effective and efficient use of supplies and services to care for patients. Non-labor expense is an area with significant opportunity for leaders to reduce unnecessary waste and expense. **Non-labor expense** accounts for 20% to 30% of healthcare provider organizations' total operating expense and includes disposable medical supplies, drugs, medical devices, and purchased services. The goal of managing non-labor productivity is to provide the right supply or service to the right patient at the right time and at the right price (Box 7.1).

BOX 7.1

GOALS OF MANAGING NON-LABOR PRODUCTIVITY

- ▪ Right supply or service
- ▪ Right patient
- ▪ Right time
- ▪ Right price

There are numerous best practice approaches leaders can apply to reduce non-labor expense, grouped into the three major opportunity categories: acquisition, utilization, and evaluation (Box 7.2). Acquisition through effective supply chain management involves the processes designed to procure, store, and distribute products and services. Utilization is the type, variety, and quantity of supplies and services used to support patient care activities. Evaluation is the continuous process to ensure supplies and services are meeting the strategic goals of the organization.

BOX 7.2

CATEGORIES OF MANAGING NON-LABOR PRODUCTIVITY
1. Acquisition
2. Utilization
3. Evaluation

ACQUISITION

Non-labor expense is largely determined by the acquisition cost of supplies and services. In most cases this critical function is driven by supply chain and contract managers who work closely with leaders to understand and fulfill their needs to support safe and high quality care. Leaders have influence in selecting which products and services are used to satisfy their and their patients' needs. Pricing is typically set through the healthcare provider organization's **group purchasing organization (GPO)** or negotiated separately.

A GPO supports healthcare provider organizations' achieving efficiency and savings by aggregating purchasing power to negotiate discounts with manufacturers, distributers, and other vendors. Optimizing the use of negotiated national GPO agreements allows leaders to access a range of products and services. Leaders may also work with other vendors when their needs cannot be met by the GPO. In which case local agreements can be negotiated. A step-by-step process for negotiating competitive pricing for supplies and services is addressed later in the chapter.

UTILIZATION

Utilization is the second area of non-labor productivity opportunity. Reducing unnecessary and costly use or overuse of supplies and services provides a significant opportunity to cut waste. Supply chain management is a critical part of providing effective and efficient care by getting the right product to the right patient at the right time. Improving non-labor productivity through utilization includes leveraging effective supply chain management tactics, using evidence-based clinical guidelines, and assessing the use of physician preference items (PPIs).

Supply Chain Management

Effective **supply chain management** includes standardizing products, maintaining adequate supply levels, enforcing drug and supply formularies, and preventing expired drugs and medical supplies. Leaders should collaborate with supply chain managers to control unnecessary inventory expense from over-stocking, not stocking the right supplies, or expired supplies that must be discarded. Consider the potential cost savings from standardizing products whenever possible to reduce the number of invoices and inventory. Implementing standard formularies that restrict staff from ordering unapproved drugs and supplies, including non-medical items such as office supplies, can control non-labor expense.

Leaders should also work closely with supply chain managers to establish, continuously assess, and adjust inventory stock known as a par level. The **par level** is the lowest stock volume that can be maintained without risking running short yet low enough to avoid costly overstocking. A common approach to managing supply levels is just in time (JIT) inventory. A **JIT inventory** model is designed to increase efficiency and reduce unnecessary expense by receiving products only as they are needed for use. The goal of JIT inventory is to have the right supplies available to meet demand without over-stocking causing higher than necessary inventory expense.

Effective supply chain management can also prevent costly expired supplies. The National Academy of Medicine[1] found that wasted medical supplies in usable condition add up to an estimated $765 billion a year in the United States. The common practice of hoarding supplies in drawers, cabinets, and lab coat pockets, especially when the par level is not maintained, leads to significant waste from expired products that need to be discarded. Engaging clinical staff to maintain adequate par levels supports making sure the right supplies are available when and where needed. Some effective techniques for preventing expired medical supplies include rotating products nearing expiration to the front for first use, clearly labeling items nearing expiration with a colorful "Use First" sticker, and moving items nearing expiration to other departments or services where they'll most likely be used.[2] Lastly, developing a quarterly expiration monitoring program with clinical and supply chain leaders will ensure all supply storage locations are checked for soon-to-expire items.

Expired medications is another opportunity for significant savings. Research shows that most medicines are effective well beyond their labeled expiration date and could be safely prescribed to patients. Despite the current limitations on prescribing expired drugs by the Food and Drug Administration, applying the Shelf Life Extension Program (SLEP) testing protocols could effectively extend the availability of expensive drugs while reducing medication shortages.[3] SLEP is a program requiring U.S. federal agencies to evaluate and extend the shelf life of stockpiled medication after undergoing stability testing to ensure the drugs are still effective and safe. The drug manufacturer can also extend the drug expiration date based on data from stability studies through approved protocols.[4]

Linen and laundry use are often ignored areas for potential cost savings. Inefficient processes that create overutilization are often embedded into workflows. Closely monitoring linen use to prevent loss and instituting a linen utilization program are two effective techniques to reduce waste.[5] Linen can often leave the healthcare provider organization through inappropriate waste disposal, with ambulance crews, and with discharged patients. Leaders should make staff mindful of the cost of waste from linen that is improperly disposed through biohazard waste and with patients. If not already in place, a linen utilization program with a multidisciplinary linen committee can introduce discipline and rigor to eliminate waste. A linen committee should review and be empowered to implement policies and procedures to support effective and efficient use of linen, including the key areas listed in Box 7.3.[6] Lastly, while healthcare provider organizations must provide certain staff with scrubs, there must be guidelines and controls in place to prevent waste through enforcing simple policies and procedures.

BOX 7.3

LINEN UTILIZATION REVIEW

- Frequency of bed changes
- Standard bed make-up
- Handling of stained, torn, or soiled linen
- Par level amount of linen in patients' rooms
- Exchange protocol with ambulance crews

A final supply chain management area to consider is disposable medical devices labeled "for single use only" that can be cleaned and safely reused at approximately half the cost of the original device.[7] Reprocessing single-use clinical devices is regulated by the FDA. Despite the controversy and misperceptions that may hinder healthcare provider organizations from reprocessing single-use clinical devices, leaders should nonetheless explore the potential benefits and risks.

Non-Labor Productivity Measurement and Analysis

Two common measures for evaluating non-labor productivity are supply costs per inpatient discharge, outpatient visit, or other unit of service (UoS) and inventory turnover. Supply costs per UoS reflects both acquisition cost and utilization. The formula for calculating supply cost per UoS is provided in Box 7.4.

BOX 7.4

CALCULATING SUPPLY COST PER UNIT OF SERVICE

$$\text{Supply cost per UoS} = \frac{\text{Total expense for UoS}}{\text{Units of service}}$$

For example, assessing the pharmacy cost per adjusted surgery for the Regional Health System's (RHS) Department of Surgical Services for FY 20X2 year-to-date (YTD) September can be calculated using the department P&L in Appendix D as follows:

$$\text{Drug expense per adjusted surgery} = \frac{\text{Total drug supply expense}}{\text{Adjusted surgeries}} = \frac{\$5,438}{2,528}$$

$$= \$2.15 \text{ drug expense per adjusted admission}$$

Recall from Chapter 4 that a single measurement in and of itself does not provide any useful comparison. For comparison, using the same formula in Box 7.4, the drug expense per adjusted surgery for FY 20X1 YTD September was $3,222. Dividing the FY 20X1 YTD drug cost by the total number of adjusted surgeries (2,038) equals $1.58 drug expense per adjusted admission. The drug cost per adjusted surgery case increased $.057 or almost 27% year over year. The specific type of variance including rate, efficiency, and volume presented in Chapter 4 will be addressed later in the case example. All of the supply or service cost per UoS measures can be case mix-adjusted to reflect changes in expense due to sicker patients.

As presented in Chapter 4, the financial asset efficiency ratio for inventory management optimization can be measured and monitored through the inventory turnover ratio shown in Box 7.5. **Inventory turnover** measures the dollars of total revenue generated by each dollar of inventory.

BOX 7.5

CALCULATING TOTAL INVENTORY TURNOVER RATIO

$$\text{Inventory turnover} = \frac{\text{Total revenue}}{\text{Inventory}}$$

For example, determining the inventory turnover rate for the RHS Department of Surgical Services for FY 20X2 YTD September is calculated as follows:

$$\text{Inventory turnover} = \frac{\$1,360,132 \text{ (total operating revenue)}}{\$325,741 \text{ (average inventory)}}$$

4.2 turns per year

Average inventory is calculated by adding beginning inventory to the ending inventory and then dividing by two. A higher inventory turnover ratio is better and indicates more efficient use of the business enterprise's inventory to generate revenue. A lower turnover implies possible excess inventory causing unnecessary expense and using limited inventory storage space that can be used for other products.

The more frequently used inventory turnover rate for leading retail organizations like Wal-Mart is 7 to 10 times per year. For best practice healthcare provider organizations, particularly those that are procedure-intensive like the operating room or cardiac catheterization lab, four to five inventory turns per year may be reasonable due to different sizes and other types of products that need to be kept on hand "just in case" to have a higher inventory rate without compromising patient safety.[8] One final consideration when assessing inventory turnover is that business enterprises may stockpile inventory prior to traditionally busy seasons to satisfy the expected stronger demand, such as flu season. Therefore, the inventory for a particular quarter should not be used to calculate inventory turnover; rather, an average inventory over a period of time is a better indication of inventory effectiveness.

Evidence-Based Clinical Guidelines

Leaders can have the greatest impact on reducing non-labor expense by setting and adhering to evidence-based usage guidelines, such as drug formularies, standard order sets, and physician preference cards to avoid commonly wasted items, including drugs, disposable medical supplies, and linen. A **standard order set** is a standing clinical order for a specific medical condition or procedure, usually within an electronic health record, that defines the care process typically including the products and services to be used. For example, a common standard physician-approved standard order is nurses administering the flu vaccine to patients. Reviewing standard order sets to make sure ordered drugs and diagnostics tests support the desired clinical outcome can be a significant opportunity to reduce waste. The two specific clinical guideline areas leaders can focus on to improve non-labor productivity are PPIs and demand matching.

Physician Preference Items

Providers' use of supplies and services should be a focal point for leaders. Most care cannot be provided without an order from a provider or advanced practice provider, such as a nurse practitioner or a physician's assistant. As the adage goes, the provider's pen (or today a keyboard) is the most expensive piece of medical equipment. **Physician preference items (PPIs)** including high-cost implantable medical devices, such as implantable cardiac devices (ICDs) and orthopedic hip and knee prosthetic implants, are driving significant spending growth. PPIs account for 30% to 40% of a healthcare provider organization's total supply expense.[9] Reducing expensive PPIs without adversely affecting clinical outcomes or jeopardizing often delicate relationships with the medical staff can be challenging and requires support from senior leaders and providers. Implementing a successful PPI initiative to improve clinical program value by improving provider choice and offering competitive pricing requires a deliberate approach, presented in Box 7.6.

BOX 7.6

FIVE STEPS FOR CONDUCTING A PHYSICIAN PREFERENCE ITEM (PPI) INITIATIVE
STEP 1. Collect and analyze data
STEP 2. Engage and communicate with physicians
STEP 3. Engage and communicate with vendors
STEP 4. Implement initiative
STEP 5. Measure, monitor, and manage

STEP 1. Data Collection and Analysis

The first step to navigating this challenging process is collecting and analyzing all available data to understand the potential impact of the initiative including aggregated cost savings. Useful data to conduct a thorough analysis include implant cost by component, physician, surgical case, and vendor. The healthcare provider organization's GPOs can provide the cost per component from other member organizations. Standard national stock numbers (NSN) for each specific component allow an appropriate comparison. The GPO should also provide comparative benchmark data to help estimate the preliminary pricing proposal and potential cost savings. The preliminary analysis should be presented to senior executive leaders for their input and buy-in prior to sharing with stakeholder providers.

STEP 2. Physician Engagement and Communication

The next and most critical step is to identify, engage, and communicate with the key provider stakeholders, particularly physicians who will be impacted by any changes. The provider communication plan should include a well-developed, brief presentation with the goals of the PPI initiative, data analysis summary, and the preliminary proposal with the identified potential cost savings from Step 1. The goal of any PPI initiative is to improve quality by making sure the clinical service or program is financially viable and sustainable.

Physician Preference Item Initiative Talking Points With Providers

The initial conversations with stakeholder physicians before any actions are taken should be low key. Leaders should not make a big deal out of the need to continuously assess opportunities to control increasing costs while mitigating any potential adverse effect on clinical outcomes. The most effective conversations take place over a casual cup of coffee, at the operating room scrub sink, or over lunch in the physicians' lounge. An example of the initial conversation:

> "Dr. Smith, I just wanted to make sure you were in the loop that we are seeking more competitive pricing from our vendors in case your rep speaks with you about it. If they do, please direct them to me so we can communicate the goals and process of the initiative. Thanks for your continued support."

Matrix Pricing

An effective approach for achieving significant cost savings without compromising quality is matrix pricing. **Matrix pricing** is an increasingly popular vendor strategy, particularly with bundled payments, that caps the price a vendor can charge for each type of implantable system, regardless of the individual component cost and based on the acuity demand match with the specific patient needs. An example of matrix pricing for "high," "medium," and "low" demand hip implants is shown in Table 7.1.

Matrix pricing is often preferred by providers who want more choices for their patients. It also avoids putting leaders in the awkward position of asking providers to use more or less of a certain type of implant based on need to achieve volume or **market-share pricing** that offers increasing discounts to the healthcare provider organization based on usage tiers. Having the implant

TABLE 7.1 Sample Matrix Pricing for Total Hip Arthroplasty (THA)

PROCEDURE	ACQUISITION COST BY TYPE (PATIENT ACUITY)		
	LOW DEMAND	MEDIUM DEMAND	HIGH DEMAND
THA (all components)	$7,500	$9,000	$10,500

delivered on consignment the day prior to surgery avoids carrying high inventory cost.

A matrix pricing approach provides a level playing field on which all vendors are allowed to play, including those not currently servicing the organization. It's important to communicate that the organization is not impacting provider choice if the vendor chooses not to participate in the matrix pricing program; rather, the vendor is choosing not to support the providers and their patients. The final matrix pricing contract with vendors should stipulate that any new technology or implantable devices introduced during the agreement term must be approved by the value analysis team (VAT), addressed later in the chapter. Engaging the provider stakeholders and maintaining positive and continuous communication throughout the process is critical for the success of the PPI initiative. Senior leaders should be involved and communicating with providers as much as possible to avoid the potential for vendors' undermining the process. Ask the providers to support the process by referring vendors who approach them to the designated organizational point of contact to avoid their being caught in the middle.

STEP 3. Vendor Engagement and Communication

After getting the providers on board the next step is to engage the vendors, those currently working with the organization and other vendors invited to participate in the process. An example of the initial communication to the vendors is provided in Exhibit 7.1. Healthcare provider organizations typically

EXHIBIT 7.1

SAMPLE INITIAL LETTER TO VENDORS

March 1, 20X3

Dear Vendor,

As I'm sure you are aware, the current and anticipated increasing regulatory and economic pressure will continue to challenge Regional Health System's financial performance and the ability to support our mission of delivering excellence in quality and service.

With these challenges in mind we will pursue innovative ways to improve clinical effectiveness while reducing our operating expense. We must work closely with our vendor partners to better align decreasing revenues with increasing operating expenses to sustain our mission.

I appreciate your commitment and support throughout this important process and value our relationship. I look forward to our continued working together.

Sincerely,

Jane Smith, Vice President, RHS

EXHIBIT 7.2

SAMPLE LETTER OF PHYSICIAN SUPPORT

March 1, 20X2

Dear Vendor,

The undersigned physicians are committed to ensuring high quality and cost-effective care at Regional Health System. In order to sustain RHS's mission we must continuously explore opportunities for improving value—both from the patient's and the payer's perspective.

We hereby fully support the efforts to work closely with our vendor partners to better align shrinking revenues with increasing operating expenses to enable clinical efficacy, efficiency, and growth.

We request and appreciate your full attention and assistance in this important initiative. Please direct any questions or concerns to Jane Smith, Vice President, RHS.

Sincerely,

Physician Names and Signatures

---

have a formal **request for proposal** (RFP) process to invite competitive pricing bids from vendors. After all vendor proposals are submitted and analyzed, meetings with vendors should be held to clarify and negotiate competitive pricing. Another important communication to share with vendors is the endorsement of the PPI initiative by stakeholder providers, shown in Exhibit 7.2. Once the vendor meetings and final negotiations are concluded, the final proposal known as the **best and final offer** (BAFO) should be shared with providers for any input or questions prior to finalizing the pricing matrix.

STEP 4. Implementation

The next important step in the PPI initiative process is implementing the negotiated savings with all participating vendors. Implementation typically involves entering all of the relevant pricing information from the new vendor agreements into the contract management system. It might also involve revising the inventory or stockage levels. There may also be a need to conduct training for employees on any new products. A sample letter announcing the final matrix pricing to the vendors is presented in Exhibit 7.3. A possible negotiating technique vendors may use is refusing to accept the final matrix pricing, in which case it's critical to communicate with providers the importance of continuing to support the initiative, including their letting the vendor know that cases could be transitioned to another vendor if they refuse to support the organization.

EXHIBIT 7.3

ANNOUNCEMENT LETTER TO VENDORS

April 1, 20X2

Dear Vendor,

We appreciate your continued commitment to high quality and service to our physicians and their patients at Regional Health System. With their full support we present the enclosed final Implant Pricing Matrix and Terms and Conditions reflecting our analysis of what other organizations are paying for the same products.

The new pricing structure is effective January 1, 20X3. Notify me no later than November 1 if you are unable to accept the pricing to allow time to make the necessary arrangements with our physicians to transition their cases to another vendor.

We look forward to working with you. Contact me directly with any questions. Thanks for your support.

Sincerely,

Jane Smith, Vice President, RHS

Enclosure

STEP 5. Measure, Monitor, and Manage

The final step is to measure, track and report, and make any necessary changes to achieve and sustain the targeted savings while continuing to monitor quality outcomes. Leveraging accurate data and maintaining strong relationships with the providers through frequent and positive communications throughout the entire process, including after implementing the new pricing matrix, are the two most critical elements to the success of a PPI initiative. Leaders should have a dashboard to monitor key performance indicators using the same data measures collected during Step 1. The achieved cost savings should be compared to the target and reported to senior leaders and stakeholder providers on a periodic basis to monitor and address any variance. One potential source of variance from the projected cost savings goal is vendors gaming the system by influencing providers' selection of the implant type. This tactic increases the total cost per case without violating the matrix pricing terms. A well-developed demand matching program can prevent this from occurring.

Demand Matching Program

Not all implantable medical devices or prosthetics are created equal. For example, the typical cost of a primary hip implant can range from $3,000 to $10,000 or more based on the technology used. The business enterprise's making or losing money on the case is largely dependent upon the implant cost.[10] While well-intended device and implant vendors seek to satisfy the needs and expectations of end-user providers and their patients, they also have a vested interest to increase profit by selling the highest priced device possible. What's more, providers may be ambivalent to the cost paid by the healthcare provider organization since it doesn't usually impact their compensation for performing the surgery. Research shows that most orthopedic surgeons are unaware of the cost of an implant.[11] With new techniques and technologies being introduced, controlling non-labor costs for PPI is dependent upon ensuring the implant matches patient need and acuity.

Demand matching is a deliberate provider-driven process to determine the most appropriate implant for each patient.[12] Demand matching can reduce unnecessary cost without compromising clinical outcomes by engaging the provider, patient, and healthcare provider organization throughout the process. For example, a relatively younger and physically active patient may require a "high-demand" hip or knee implant versus a bed-bound older patient who will have a good outcome with a lower demand implant. An effective demand matching program uses an objective evidence-based clinical algorithm to remove any potential for bias or vendor influence.

EVALUATION

The final area of non-labor productivity management is evaluation. Leaders should be involved with formally and continuously evaluating all products and services to ensure they meet the highest standards of safety, quality, and service at the lowest possible price. What's more, leaders should work closely with vendors to identify and monetize the clinical efficacy of their products and services to create sustainable strategic partnerships. There are three interrelated components of evaluation: value analysis for new products and services, purchased service analysis for existing vendor relationships, and value partnering for creating sustainable strategic vendor relationships.

Value Analysis Process

As new products, services, and technology are continuously introduced leaders must have a formal process to measure, assess, balance, and prioritize both clinical efficacy and cost efficiency. The purpose and goal of the **value analysis process (VAP)** is to promote key stakeholder and end-user input to product and service decisions based on quality, safety, and value. Providers and other clinicians should be actively engaged in the VAP. Data analytics is a key component to an effective VAP to identify and leverage ongoing opportunities. Figure 7.1 provides a sample VAP.[13]

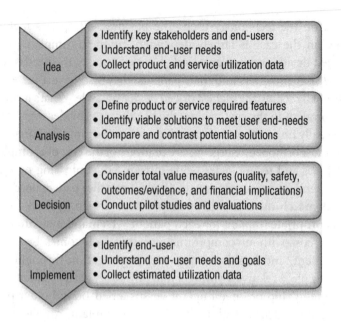

FIGURE 7.1 Value analysis process.

A critical part of the VAP is leaders forming, engaging, and participating in **value analysis teams (VATs)** that are empowered to make decisions to identify and reconcile quality and cost with both current and new products and services. VATs are critical to the success of the VAP and are typically formed at a steering or specialty or service line level, such as surgery, cardiovascular, or diagnostic imaging. The role and responsibilities of a VAT are threefold, summarized in Box 7.7.

BOX 7.7

ROLE AND RESPONSIBILITIES OF THE VALUE ANALYSIS TEAM (VAT)

1. Assess new and existing products and services
2. Identify acceptable solutions and substitutes
3. Review new item or service requests

The VAT should review product or service categories for standardization and utilization savings opportunities, including those that allow for greater GPO contract compliance as long as clinical needs are met. Next, the VAT should proactively create clinically acceptable substitution lists for critical products rather than wait for a backorder or recall. The final role of the VAT is to review all new item requests. New products or services should not be introduced to the organization without VAT review and approval. This includes specialty nursing, such as wound care or infection prevention, and all PPIs. Patient care and safety dictate the need for an exception to VAT approval on a case-by-case basis. As new items and services are added to the inventory, the healthcare provider organization must have a process in place to monitor, review, and assess their performance.

Purchased Services Analysis

Healthcare provider organizations contract with vendors to provide an array of products and services, both patient and non-patient care related. In some cases the organization is unable to produce the services offered by vendors, such as blood banking and external auditing. Leaders should evaluate the trade-offs between providing services internally (**insourcing**) and contracting with a vendor (**outsourcing**) based on which option can provide the highest quality at the lowest price. The steps for conducting a make (insource) versus buy (outsource) analysis to assess the financial impact of providing a service internally or contracting with an external vendor are addressed in Box 7.8.

The decision to insource or outsource is usually strategic and often financially driven. Among the key reasons to consider providing a service internally are that there is no other viable option, organizational capacity exists, or there is a need for direct control over the service. The primary reasons for considering outsourcing include a lack of internal expertise or capacity, quality or service challenges, and regulatory compliance needs. A step-by-step process for evaluating the decision to insource or outsource is presented in Box 7.8.

BOX 7.8

STEPS FOR ASSESSING INSOURCING VS. OUTSOURCING OPPORTUNITIES

STEP 1. Conduct a comprehensive inventory of all purchased services including annual expense by category and expiration date. See Appendix F for a Purchased Services Inventory Checklist.

STEP 2. Interview key clinical and operational end-user representatives to collect feedback on service performance.

STEP 3. Develop decision-making and evaluation criteria, including quality, safety, reliability, service, and financial measures.

STEP 4. Identify and prioritize opportunities to insource or outsource.

(continued)

BOX 7.8 (continued)

STEP 5. Initiate a formal RFP process.
STEP 6. Organize and conduct vendor negotiations.
STEP 7. Develop and implement action plans based on prioritized opportunities.
STEP 8. Coordinate with external partners, including GPOs and vendors, to facilitate purchased service transitions.
STEP 9. Facilitate employee training for any new services.
STEP 10. Hardwire contract savings into the enterprise resource management system.

Strategic Value Partnering

To survive in a value-based care environment where reimbursement is based on demonstrating value rather than the volume of services delivered, healthcare provider organizations must develop strategic, mutually beneficial, and sustainable partnerships with key vendors. Vendors seeking to partner with healthcare provider organizations are under increasing pressure to add value beyond highly reliable products and services, where value is quality divided by cost. Most vendors can articulate how they improve quality through their value proposition; however, many struggle with understanding and quantifying cost and return on investment from the healthcare provider organization's perspective. At the same time, healthcare provider organizations are challenged with monetizing value by connecting the vendor's proposal to the anticipated financial impact. Healthcare provider organizations should seek strategic partnerships with key vendors beyond a transactional relationship by defining and quantifying both the quality and the financial impact of the vendor's proposal and then sharing risk on the planned outcome benefit. A good litmus test for evaluating a potential strategic partnership with vendors is asking two simple and direct questions, shown in Box 7.9.

BOX 7.9

STRATEGIC PARTNERSHIP TEST: TWO QUESTIONS TO ASK A VENDOR

1. *Will the product or service achieve the simultaneous goals of improving quality and reducing cost?*
2. *Assuming it will, are you willing to share financial risk in the outcome?*

Ultimately both partners in a mutually beneficial relationship should have some skin in the game such that their interests are closely aligned. Quantifying the projected financial return through a well-defined business case is addressed in Chapter 9.

REGIONAL HEALTH SYSTEM CASE EXAMPLE: REDUCING NON-LABOR EXPENSE

The Director of Surgical Services continued her assessment of opportunities to reduce unnecessary operating expense identified in the financial condition analysis in Chapter 4 and the variance analysis addressed in Chapter 5. After completing her review, identification, and implementation of labor productivity opportunities, she turned her attention to non-labor productivity initiatives, including reducing expired drugs and medical supplies, switching to lower cost supplies, using fewer supplies, and decreasing linen and scrub use. The RHS CFO asked the Director to quantify and annualize all of her projected labor expense savings for the next fiscal year (FY 20X3). The variance analysis conducted by the Director presented in Chapter 5 identified an opportunity to reduce medical supply cost. The unfavorable rate, efficiency, and volume variances contributed to the $44,502 total non-labor variance for September FY 20X2 shown in Exhibit 7.4. The non-labor variance for the YTD FY 20X2 provided in Appendix D for the department is $92,845.

EXHIBIT 7.4

MONTHLY NON-LABOR EXPENSE DETAIL FOR REGIONAL HEALTH SYSTEM'S DEPARTMENT OF SURGICAL SERVICES

	SEPTEMBER FY 20X2			
MEDICAL SUPPLIES	**ACTUAL**	**BUDGET**	**VARIANCE**	**% VARIANCE**
Medical supply cost	$223,896	$179,394	$(44,502)	−24.8%
Units of supply	2,231	2,000	(231)	−11.6%
UNITS OF SERVICE (UoS)				
Procedures (adjusted)	699	670	29	4.3%
Supply cost per unit	$100.36	$89.70	$(10.66)	−11.9%
Supplies per UoS	3.19	2.99	(0.21)	−6.9%

Switching to Lower Cost Supplies and Using Fewer Supplies

In collaboration with supply chain managers and the GPO to better match supply needs and achieve more competitive pricing, the Director anticipates being able to reduce medical supply cost. At the same time she worked closely with clinical leaders to reduce medical supply utilization by revising clinical order sets with built-in waste. The savings from eliminating the need for or replacing supplies with lower cost alternatives is easy to calculate by subtracting the projected cost with the implemented changes from the historical cost. Switching from a local vendor to a GPO vendor with a lower contracted price for surgical gowns, masks, and latex gloves, the Director expects to save $17,572 annually calculated as follows:

Medical and surgical supply costs for FY 20X2: (surgical gowns, masks, and latex gloves)	$133,681
Medical and surgical supply costs for FY 20X3: (estimated based on projected volume)	−$116,109
Projected annual cost savings:	$17,572

Preventing Expired Medical Supplies and Drugs

Implementing the supply chain management techniques previously presented, the Director expects to decrease expired drugs and medical supplies saving the department an estimated $37,550 per year. The projected savings was estimated by collecting and monetizing expired, unusable medical supplies over a month's period and then annualizing the amount. The Director created awareness among her staff by putting the expired medical supplies in a large box and labeling it with the total cost of waste.

Decreasing Linen and Scrub Use

As part of an organization-wide initiative to control linen and scrub expense, the Director was asked to represent the Department of Surgical Services on the RHS Linen Committee. Among the planned actions to reduce an estimated $3,016 in annual expense savings is maintaining adequate linen par levels to avoid needing to process clean linen, implementing a scrub control policy, and working with the linen and laundry vendor to adopt best practices for reducing expense.

The total projected annual cost savings opportunity for FY 20X3 resulting from the Director's non-labor productivity initiatives is $58,138, summarized in Table 7.2.

TABLE 7.2 **Planned Non-Labor Expense Initiatives and Projected Financial Impact**

NON-LABOR EXPENSE REDUCTION INITIATIVE	FINANCIAL IMPACT
1. Negotiate more competitive contract pricing and revise clinical order sets to reduce medical supply expense by 13%.	$17,572
2. Adopt effective supply chain management tactics to decrease expired drug and medical supplies expense.	$37,550
3. Implement linen and scrub utilization controls.	$3,016
Total projected annual non-labor expense reduction	$58,138

SUMMARY

Leaders accountable for the financial and operations performance of their business enterprise must continuously assess opportunities to improve the safety, quality, and efficiency of the products and services provided to their patients. The goal of improving non-labor productivity is to get the right supply or service to the right patient at the right time and at the right price. Leaders can use the VAP, purchased services analysis, PPI initiative, and demand matching to exercise discipline, control, oversight, and clinical and administrative team collaboration to improve non-labor productivity and reduce expense.

CALLS TO ACTION

Leaders should:

- Recognize the significant impact improving non-labor productivity has on reducing operating expense to achieve financial performance goals.
- Implement proven effective tactics for improving non-labor productivity, including a physician preference initiative and demand matching program.
- Collaborate with supply chain leaders to continuously assess product and service efficacy and efficiency through strategic vendor relationships, including value analysis, purchased services analysis, and value partnering.

References

1. Institute of Medicine National Academy of Medicine. Best care at lower cost: the path to continuously learning health care in America. Report Brief. 2012. https://nam.edu/wp-content/uploads/2017/12/Briefing-Book_Combined.pdf

2. DateCheck Pro for Healthcare. The quick-guide to healthcare expiration date management: best practices for training materials handling staff. https://www.datecheckhealth.com/wp-content/uploads/dlm_uploads/2018/06/Healthcare-Quick-Guide-to-Expiration-Date-Management.pdf

3. Diven DG, Bartenstein DW, Carroll DR. Extending shelf life just makes sense. *Mayo Clin Proc.* 2015;90(1):1471-1474. https://www.mayoclinicproceedings.org/article/S0025-6196(15)00667-9/abstract.

4. U.S. Food & Drug Administration. Expiration dating extension. https://www.fda.gov/emergency-preparedness-and-response/mcm-legal-regulatory-and-policy-framework/expiration-dating-extension

5. Vizient. Follow the linen to reduce the money trail. November 13, 2018. https://newsroom.vizientinc.com/newsletter/research-and-insights-news/follow-linen-reduce-money-trail

6. Becker's Healthcare. Washing out unnecessary linen costs. Hospital CFO Report. November 6, 2015. https://www.beckershospitalreview.com/finance/washing-out-unnecessary-linen-costs.html

7. Lagasse J. Reprocessing medical devices can result in significant savings for hospitals. Healthcare Finance. February 20, 2019. https://www.healthcarefinancenews.com/news/reprocessing-medical-devices-can-result-significant-savings-hospitals

8. Mobile Aspects. The key inventory management metric for hospitals to track. August 23, 2018. https://www.mobileaspects.com/the-key-inventory-management-metric-for-hospitals-to-track/

9. Pettigrew P, Fiedler B, Jehle B. Leveling the playing field in physician preference items. *Healthcare Financial Management.* 2013.

10. American Association of Hip and Knee Surgeons. Total joint replacement: a breakdown of costs. https://hipknee.aahks.org/total-joint-replacement-a-breakdown-of-costs/

11. Okike K, O'Toole RV, Pollak AN, et al. Survey finds few orthopedic surgeons know the costs of the devices they implant. *Health Aff.* 2014;33(1):103-109. https://www.healthaffairs.org/doi/full/10.1377/hlthaff.2013.0453

12. O'Donnell E, Alvarez LO. Demand matching: balancing cost and quality to maximize greatest postoperative outcomes. *J Health Care Finance.* 2006;33(2):1-5.

13. Meyers Janda C. *Supply Chain Value and Non-labor Expense Management.* University of Minnesota, School of Public Health Presentation; 2011.

CHAPTER 8

GROWING PROFITABLE VOLUME AND MARKET SHARE

Incidence rate	Secret shopping
Prevalence rate	Herfindahl-Hirschman Index (HHI)
Capacity	Competitive differentiation
Competitor analysis	Service recovery
Competitor	Value proposition

INTRODUCTION

Incremental revenue generated from volume growth is the lifeblood of any healthcare provider organization. Healthcare provider organizations cannot shrink their way to prosperity by focusing primarily on cost cutting measures. Increasing profitable market share supports an organization's strategic goals such as investing in patient safety and quality improvement initiatives, expanding ambulatory capacity, offering new programs and services to support community need, acquiring the latest medical technology to stay competitive, and recruiting qualified providers and staff. Volume and revenue targets are typically developed during the annual budgeting process covered in Chapter 3. Leaders must continuously develop, implement, and monitor comprehensive growth plans to support the organization's mission and achieve its strategic and financial performance goals.

DEVELOPING THE FIVE-STEP BLUEPRINT FOR GROWTH

Comprehensive growth planning includes several important assessment needs. Leaders must first understand their market including the current and projected population and demographic trends that will affect the type and amount of services needed to support accurate demand forecasting. Projecting future volume allows leaders to determine if they have sufficient capacity to adequately handle the anticipated incremental volume or if they need to add resources, such as providers, staff, and space. Leaders must then evaluate other organizations in their market to understand how they can differentiate their services through a well-defined value proposition. Lastly, leaders should have a plan for how they can leverage the market growth opportunities identified during the planning process. The framework presented in Box 8.1 provides a step-by-step approach leaders can use to grow profitable volume and market share.

STEP 1. Define and Assess the Market

The first step in growing profitable volume is to define and assess the market in which the healthcare provider organization operates. A **market** is an actual

---

BOX 8.1

FIVE-STEP BLUEPRINT FOR GROWTH
STEP 1. Define and assess the market.
STEP 2. Forecast demand.
STEP 3. Identify and assess competitors.
STEP 4. Define the value proposition.
STEP 5. Develop and implement the growth plan.

---

or virtual place where the organization interacts with its customers or patients directly or through intermediaries, such as a provider acting as an agent for patients. A market is comprised of both current patients and potential customers. Patients and customers are different even though the terms are used interchangeably. A patient is currently receiving healthcare services while a customer is a potential, future patient. A market includes patients who have accessed services from the business enterprise within a specified time period, typically a year.

The healthcare provider organization's **primary service area (PSA)** is a geographic zone defined by the zip codes, usually contiguous or connecting, that comprise 75% to 80% of its patients based on where they live. A **secondary service area (SSA)** is comprised of the remaining 20% to 25% of its patients. Figure 8.1 presents a sample map identifying the PSA and SSA for a specific geographic market. The organization's total service area is commonly referred as a catchment area. Besides location, patients and customers can be grouped into sub-categories according to similar traits known as a market segment.

Market Segmentation

A **market segment** is a sub-set of patients or customers who share one or more common characteristics. Segmenting a market is useful to support identifying, planning for, and delivering services that meet patients' needs and expectations. For example, the healthcare services required by a 65-year-old female retiree will be different than those needed by a family of six with school-aged children. There are several categories of market segments shown in Box 8.2.

Where patients live is an important consideration for what type of healthcare services should be offered and where they should be located. Most patients prefer to receive care closer to home, usually within a 15-minute drive. Patients requiring more specialized care or highly loyal patients will typically drive 30 minutes or longer.[1] Markets can be segmented by specific demographics including age, gender, race, ethnicity, education, income, and employment status.

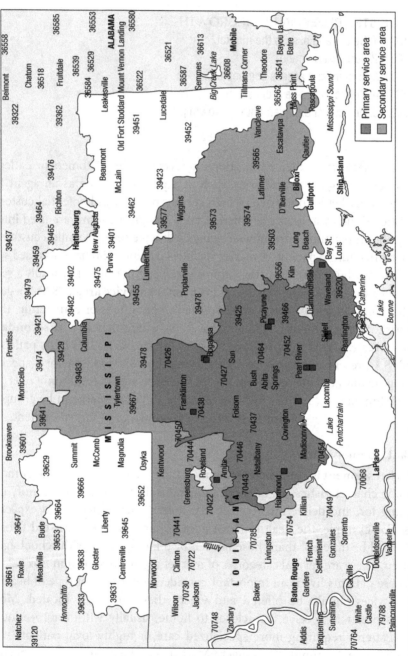

FIGURE 8.1 Primary and secondary service area map example.

BOX 8.2

TYPES OF MARKET SEGMENTS
- Geographic
- Demographic
- Clinical service
- Payer

Patients can also be grouped according to their specific clinical care needs, such as by service line or disease state, for example cardiovascular, musculoskeletal, women, and children. Patients can also be grouped according to their eligibility to receive certain insurance benefits, such as Medicare or by type of employer. For example, a market segment comprised of large manufacturing firms may require more occupational health and industrial medicine services. Understanding the specific populations served by the healthcare provider organization through market segmentation allows leaders to conduct an effective demand analysis, the next step in developing the blueprint for growth.

STEP 2. Forecast Demand

Accurately forecasting future patient volume through a demand analysis is essential for efficient resource planning and effective service delivery. A **demand analysis** is a deliberate process to forecast patient volumes within a specified service and time frame. Effective demand forecasting also takes the guesswork out of planning for additional capacity needs, such as providers and staff, space, equipment, supplies, and services. Demand forecasting supports closing any disparities that often exist among at-risk populations through identifying and addressing social determinants of health needs such as housing, transportation, and access to healthy food.

Demand forecasting informs the annual budgeting process and reduces the need to address operating and financial variances using the process presented in Chapter 3. However, the same challenges inherent to the budgeting process also affect volume forecasting, such as unpredictable market volatility or seasonal variation. Other factors that can affect the forecasting process that must be considered include shifts in consumer demand, increased competition, advances in practice or technology, and changes in payer reimbursement.

Conducting a Demand Analysis

There are four key steps to conducting a formal demand analysis presented in Box 8.3. First the specific market segment for which the demand is to be projected must be identified. Then the market segment current and projected utilization rates must be determined. Determining projected utilization of the anticipated services needed requires a reasonably accurate assessment to assess if the current or planned capacity is adequate to handle the anticipated patient load increase. The timeline of the analysis considers the planning horizon required to estimate patient volume.

BOX 8.3

STEPS FOR CONDUCTING A DEMAND ANALYSIS
STEP 2.1. Identify market segment.
STEP 2.2. Determine utilization.
STEP 2.3. Assess capacity.
STEP 2.4. Set timeline.

STEP 2.1. Identify Market Segment

The first step in conducting a demand analysis is determining the specific market. Recall that market segments can be based on a geographic service area, demographic characteristic such as age or gender, a clinical specialty or service line, or by type of payer. The number of people living in a certain zip code and the common demographic data can be obtained through publicly available information, such as from the U.S. Census Bureau or purchased through a private data vendor. An example of how this type of data can be used to examine a specific market segment is provided in Exhibit 8.1. For example, the high-level data analysis for zip code 70437 (Folsom) shows the percent of the population aged 65 years and older and those healthcare provider organization potential customers who will be aging into Medicare within the next one to five years. Understanding the total population by demographic category is useful in determining utilization, the next step of the demand analysis.

STEP 2.2. Determine Utilization

Most healthcare provider organizations rely primarily on internal historical patient volume utilization data and trends to project future demand. Assessing historical patient utilization by service and zip code is a simple approach that can be useful to help identify population trends and make reasonable volume growth estimates. For example, the data presented in Table 8.1 show the total population in several key zip codes identified for potential growth by the organization. Several cities experienced significant growth in the primary care

EXHIBIT 8.1

SAMPLE DEMOGRAPHIC DATA BY ZIP CODE

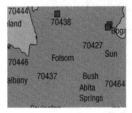

Zip Code (City)	70437 (Folsom)
Total Population	7,918
Female Population	4.067 (51.4%)
55 to 59 years	347 (4.4%)
60 to 64 years	307 (3.9%)
65 to 85 years	614 (8.6%)
Male Population	3,851 (48.6%)
55 to 59 years	323 (4.1%)
60 to 64 years	297 (3.8%)
65 to 85 years	614 (7.8%)

Source: U.S. Census Bureau, 2010 Census. www.census.gov

TABLE 8.1 **Volume Utilization Trend Example (New Patient Visits, FY 20X2–FY 20X3)**

ZIP CODE	CITY	TOTAL POPULA-TION	NEW PATIENT VISITS			
			FY 20X2	FY 20X3	VARIANCE	% VARIANCE
70437	Folsom	7,918	1,263	1,414	151	10.68%
70435	Covington	22,048	2,695	2,809	114	4.06%
70438	Franklinton	20,512	1,755	1,638	−117	−7.14%
70446	Loranger	6,835	993	1,096	103	9.40%

Source: U.S. Census Bureau, 2010 Census. www.census.gov

clinic visits from residents in several of the zip codes in the most recent year compared to the previous year.

Utilization volume trends alone, however, are not sufficient to reasonably estimate and plan for potential healthcare service needs, especially considering potential future shifts in population demographics. Is the cause of the increased patient volume variance due to population shifts, changes in service patterns, exit of a competitor, or some other reason? These questions are addressed through the formal demand analysis.

Other data besides population size, demographics, and historical patient volumes can be used to identify demand trends including service and case mix, payer mix, and inpatient versus outpatient mix to enable better accuracy and prioritization of growth opportunities. Both public and private data can be

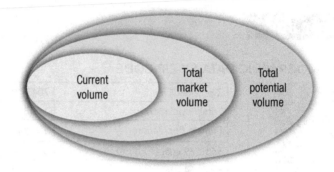

FIGURE 8.2 Identifying total potential market volume.

collected to develop a clear picture of the market or a specific market segment to support effective planning. When considering a potential capital investment for expanding existing services or adding new services to a market, two additional pieces of data are essential to accurately estimate potential incremental volume: total current market volume and total potential market volume, as illustrated in Figure 8.2.

Current volume is the organization's historical amount of services provided over a set time period, also referred to as market share. Total market volume includes all patient care delivered by the healthcare provider organization and its competitors. Patient volume data from competing organizations in the same service area can sometimes be gathered from an organization's public annual report; however, it may be too general or outdated to be useful. The most accurate and current market business intelligence, including competitor volume data, is typically purchased through third-party sources. "All payer" data reports include inpatient volume, outpatient procedures, and outpatient visits by diagnosis or procedural code, attending physician, and the site of service or location where the service was performed, such as a hospital or an ambulatory surgery center.

The total potential volume in a service area is all of the possible patient care that could be delivered in the specified market based on the projected health needs of the population including preventive, diagnostic, primary, specialty, emergent, acute, and post-acute care. **Population health management** is a holistic approach to improving health outcomes for a specific group as part of the movement toward value-based care. Understanding and identifying the population health needs of customers in a market or market segment who have not sought care is more involved, but necessary to enable leaders to assess the bigger picture for strategic resource planning and business development. Population health data for a service area are valuable for determining the type and amount of services required to care for a specified population including birth and death rates and the incidence and prevalence of common diseases. Incidence and prevalence rates are most useful for service line planning, especially for determining total market volume.

Incidence is a measure to determine a person's probability of being diagnosed with a disease during a given period of time. Incidence is the number of newly diagnosed cases of a disease. An **incidence rate** is calculated by dividing the number of new cases of a disease by the number of persons at risk for the disease, as shown in Box 8.4.

BOX 8.4

CALCULATING INCIDENCE RATE

$$\frac{\text{Number of new cases of a disease}}{\text{Total population at risk for disease}} \times 100$$

As an example of how to apply the formula for calculating incidence rate, if over the course of one year 5 women are diagnosed with breast cancer out of a total female study population of 200 who do not have breast cancer at the beginning of the study period, then the incidence of breast cancer in this population is calculated as follows:

$$\text{Incidence rate for breast cancer} = \frac{5}{200} \times 100 = 2.5 \text{ or } 2{,}500 \text{ women per } 100{,}000 \text{ women-years of study}$$

Prevalence on the other hand is a measure to determine a person's likelihood of having the disease. The number of prevalent cases is the total number of cases of disease existing in a population. The **prevalence rate** is the total number of cases of a disease existing in a population divided by the total population, shown in Box 8.5.

BOX 8.5

CALCULATING PREVALENCE RATE

$$\frac{\text{Total number of cases of a disease}}{\text{Total population (same period)}} \times 100$$

To illustrate how to calculate the prevalence rate, if a measurement of lung cancer is taken in a population of 40,000 people with 1,200 who were recently diagnosed with lung cancer and 3,500 living with cancer, then the prevalence of cancer is calculated as follows:

Prevalence rate for lung cancer = $\dfrac{4,700}{40,000} \times 100 = 11.75$ or 11,750 per 100,000 persons

Table 8.2 shows an excerpt example of the prevalence of heart disease by age, race, and gender from research published by the Centers for Disease Control and Prevention (CDC).[2]

TABLE 8.2 **Cardiac Disease Prevalence Example**

CHARACTER-ISTIC	NUMBER OF RESPON-DENTS	HEART ATTACK (%)	HEART DISEASE (%)	HEART ATTACK OR HEART DISEASE (%)
Age (years)				
18-44	128,328	0.8	1.1	1.6
45-64	137,738	4.8	5.4	7.7
≥65	87,351	12.9	13.1	19.6
Sex				
Male	136,201	5.5	5.5	8.2
Female	219,911	2.9	3.4	5.0
Race/Ethnicity				
White, non-Hispanic	279,419	4.0	4.2	6.2
Black, non-Hispanic	27,925	4.1	3.7	6.2
Asian	5,974	2.9	3.3	4.7
Hispanic	25,539	3.6	5.0	6.9
American Indian/Alaska Native	5,535	7.4	7.2	11.2
Multiracial	6,519	6.4	5.4	9.0
Education				
Less than high school diploma	38,202	6.0	6.4	9.8
High school graduate	109,830	4.5	4.5	6.8
Some college	93,228	3.9	4.5	6.4
College graduate	113,944	2.9	3.6	5.0
Total	356,112	4.0	4.4	6.5

This type of historical prevalence data is typically available by state and region and can be applied to estimate the presence of a specific disease regardless if it is diagnosed or being treated in a specific market by extrapolating the percentages of disease for each demographic category relative to proportion of the demographic living in the service area.

STEP 2.3. Assess Capacity

Capacity is the total amount of patient volume that can be handled given the desired access and service standards, such as how long on average a patient should wait to be seen in an outpatient clinic after requesting an appointment. Recommended service and access standards are addressed later. Conducting a formal **capacity analysis** can identify the need for creating additional capacity to handle more patients based on the number, type, and competency of providers and staff available, physical space and layout, workflow processes, and equipment, supplies, and services, as presented in Box 8.6. Assessing the potential demand for a business enterprise within a market segment or service area is pointless without having a clear understanding of the potential capacity needs relative to any current or potential growth constraints. Attempting to grow volume and market share without the necessary capacity could lead to dissatisfied patients and ultimately fewer patients due to their outmigrating to competitors.

BOX 8.6

CAPACITY CONSIDERATIONS
1. Providers
2. Staff
3. Physical space and layout
4. Workflow processes
5. Equipment, supplies, and services

Physical space such as the number of hospital beds or clinic exam rooms, the number and types of providers, and the staff available are critical to consider for assessing capacity. Most important and often overlooked is the capacity constraint due to poorly designed and inefficient processes that limit throughput. Finally, available and relevant labor productivity benchmarks can be used to calculate additional capacity required to adequately handle more patient volume. For example, using the average total scan, processing, and interpretation times for a diagnostic MRI can provide the number of productive labor hours required per unit of service.

Among the potential indicators for assessing capacity, wait lists or the known backlog of patients for a particular service is a clear indication of volume constraint and should be considered during the growth planning process. Healthcare provider organizations often track other inpatient and outpatient metrics to assess capacity, such as occupancy rate, operating room block time utilization, third available appointment for ambulatory care, and left without being seen (LWOBS) in the emergency department. While there is no broad agreement, the rule of thumb across various industries is that production of a particular good or service is fully utilized or at full capacity between 80% and 90%[3] to allow the necessary slack for fluctuating volume variability and avoid bottlenecks that can create dissatisfied patients and drive away business. Leaders are challenged with balancing access and service standards with volume capacity constraints and financial performance goals.

STEP 2.4. Set Timeline

The last step in conducting an effective demand analysis is determining how long the volume forecast will be relevant for the intended purpose. The predictive value of the assumptions and projections in a demand analysis can vary from 1 to 5 years depending on the dynamics and demographics of the population upon which the forecast is made. If the population size and demographic characteristics, such as employment and income, are relatively stable the projections could be used for a longer period. In any case, leaders should continuously monitor the available population demographic and health data to enable proactive planning to meet the needs of the market or market segment served.

STEP 3. Identify and Assess Competitors (Competitor Analysis)

The increasingly competitive healthcare landscape can negatively affect an organization's ability to sustain its mission as the movement to value-based care continues, forcing organizations to grow volume and market share just to sustain their current portfolio of services. To achieve strategic and financial growth goals leaders must continuously identify and systematically assess market competitors to delineate how their organization can better meet customers' needs and expectations through a formal **competitor analysis**. The goals of a competitor analysis include forecasting competitors' future strategies and decisions, predicting their likely reactions to an organization's strategy and competitive initiatives, and determining how competitors' behavior can be influenced to the benefit of the initiating organization.

A **competitor** is a business enterprise that produces the same or similar services to the healthcare provider organization within the same market. The three categories of competitors are direct, indirect, and future. Direct competitors are organizations that offer identical or similar products in the healthcare provider organization's market and typically represent the greatest competitive threat. For example, two hospitals providing comprehensive cancer services are direct competitors for the same type of patients. Indirect competitors in the provider healthcare organization's market offer similar but not the exact same services. Indirect competitors likely target markets with the same or a similar value proposition as the healthcare provider organization. Lastly, future competitors are not yet in the healthcare provider organization's market but could eventually enter to provide rival services, including disruptive innovation. For example, a new provider of virtual office visits enters the market, avoiding the common inconveniences of driving, parking, and waiting.

Competitor Analysis

As stated, a **competitor analysis** is used to identify and assess rival organizations in the healthcare provider organization's market. The competitor analysis grid shown in Exhibit 8.2 provides a comprehensive and systematic way to assess and compare market competitors' strengths and weaknesses. The grid can be completed with available quantitative data and subjective qualitative information. The same evaluative criteria are applied to the leader's organization and all competitors in the market to calculate a score that can be used as a measure for assessing how the business enterprise is positioned to grow profitable volume and market share.

After identifying the service or business enterprise that will be compared, the evaluation criteria must be chosen and weighted according to their relative

---

EXHIBIT 8.2

COMPETITOR ANALYSIS GRID EXAMPLE

COMPETITIVE CRITERIA	BUSINESS ENTERPRISE	COMPETITOR 1	COMPETITOR 2	COMPETITOR 3
1. Financial condition				
2. Access				
3. Service				
4. Quality				
5. Cost				
6. Other				

importance to customers. Assigning a score for each competitor in the absence of timely and valid numerical data to complete the grid's subjective or best-guess opinions should incorporate several key stakeholders' independent input to provide a more reliable assessment. A suggested key is provided in Table 8.3 to help translate subjective values into a scoreable measure to be compared among the healthcare provider organization and its competitors. A range of "high," "medium," and "low" or "best," "average," and "worst" can be assigned to each competitive variable that can then be quantified by assigning a number to each.

The specific performance measures used to evaluate and compare the competitive effectiveness of the healthcare provider organization must be relevant to the market. Table 8.4 provides sample evaluation criteria and data sources.

An organization's financial condition presented in Chapter 4 relates its ability to meet both short-term operating expense obligations and invest in long-term growth needs. Typically organizations struggling to meet their financial obligations are also challenged with investing in long-term growth to achieve a competitive advantage in the market.

Access to care is a strong driver of patient volume growth. For certain commoditized services, such as diagnostic imaging, patients may be willing to switch from their traditional healthcare provider organization to one that can see them faster.

Conducting **secret shopping** by calling competitors to inquire how long it would take to be seen for a specific type of need is useful information. Secret shopping provides an important source of information to understand how the business enterprise is competing based on access and service. Criteria for secret shopping are presented in Table 8.5 to consistently evaluate access and service of competitors and the healthcare provider organization. Data can be entered in time units, such as number of days for the third available appointment or the number of minutes it took to make the appointment. A numerical scale such as "1" for worst and "5" for best can be used for subjective criteria; for example, the friendliness of the scheduler. A sample secret shopping script is provided in Appendix G.

Service and quality criteria include both quantitative, publicly available reports, and subjective or anecdotal qualitative information, which can also be a reliable source. Combined these provide an accurate competitor assessment.

TABLE 8.3 **Translating Competitor Analysis Evaluation**

CRITERIA	SCORE (UNWEIGHTED)
Not applicable	0
Worst	1
Average	2
Best	3

TABLE 8.4 Competitor Analysis Evaluation Criteria and Data Sources

COMPETITIVE CRITERIA	EVALUATION MEASURE	DATA SOURCES
1. Financial condition	• Operating margin • Market share	AHD[a], MedPAR[b], bond rating agency public disclosures, certificate of need (CON) filings
2. Access to care	• Ease of making an appointment (online access, time and steps required) • Time to be seen (clinic appointment)	Secret shopping, consumer reports
3. Service	• Comprehensive services (one-stop shop) • Convenience (location, parking) • Driving distance from major population centers (highways, traffic, construction) • Patient experience	Competitor web site Direct observation Route mapping HCAHPS/CG-CAHPS[c]
4. Quality	• Clinical core measures outcomes • Reputation (perception of quality) • Facilities updated and clean	Hospital Compare[d] Public news reports, anecdotal information
5. Cost	• Charge data master (fee schedule)	Competitor web site
6. Other	• Leadership (availability, competency and continuity) • Employee satisfaction (moral, vacancies, voluntary turnover)	Public news reports, competitor web site anecdotal information

COMPETITOR DATA SOURCES:

a. American Hospital Directory (AHD): www.ahd.com.
b. Medicare Provider Analysis and Review (MedPAR): https://www.cms.gov/Research-Statistics -Data-and-Systems/Files-for-Order/LimitedDataSets/MEDPARLDSHospitalNational.
c. Hospital Consumer Assessment of Healthcare (HCAHPS): https://www.medicare.gov/hospital compare/Data/Overview.html and CGCAHPS (Clinician and Group Survey): https://cahpsdata base.ahrq.gov/cahpsidb/.
d. Hospital Compare: https://www.medicare.gov/hospitalcompare/search.html?

TABLE 8.5 Secret Shopping Criteria

EVALUATION CRITERIA	BUSINESS ENTERPRISE	COMPETITOR 1	COMPETITOR 2
1. Appointment availability (third)			
2. Time to make appointment			
3. Number of phone transfers			
4. Friendliness of scheduler			
5. Evening and weekend appointments			

The requirement for healthcare provider organizations to publicly disclose their fee schedules is largely irrelevant unless the patient is paying cash since the negotiated rates with commercial payers are confidential and usually substantially less than the published fee schedule. However, relatively higher competitor fee schedules combined with lower quality scores provides an opportunity to leverage more business from commercial payers and large employers in the market. Other criteria that can be used to objectively evaluate the organization versus its competitors include leadership capability and employee satisfaction.

Beyond identifying and comparing individual competitors, leaders should be interested in the overall competitiveness of a market when assessing the potential for adding or expanding services or possibly exiting a market due to continued financial losses due to too much competition for the same business. A common measure of market concentration is the **Herfindahl-Hirschman Index (HHI)** or HHI score primarily used by economists, though also useful for healthcare leaders. The HHI score is calculated by squaring the market share of each firm competing in the service area and then summing the resulting numbers as shown in the formula in Box 8.7. The index can range from close to zero to 10,000. The smaller the index or score the greater the competition in the market.

To illustrate an application of the HHI assume the leadership for a healthcare provider organization is considering expanding services in two service areas, each with three different organizations, and wants to gauge the level of competition in each market. The market share for the healthcare provider organizations in each service are listed in Table 8.6.

BOX 8.7

CALCULATING HERFINDAHL-HIRSCHMAN INDEX (HHI)

$HHI = (\text{provider A market share})^2 + (\text{provider B market share})^2 + (\text{provider C market share})^2\ldots$

TABLE 8.6 Calculating Herfindahl-Hirschman Index (HHI) Example

HEALTHCARE PROVIDER ORGANIZATION	MARKET SHARE	
	MARKET 1	MARKET 2
A	40%	50%
B	30%	40%
C	30%	10%
Total	100%	100%

$$\text{HHI (Market 1)} = (.40)^2 + (.30)^2 + (.30)^2 = 0.34$$

$$\text{HHI (Market 2)} = (.50)^2 + (.40)^2 + (.10)^2 = 0.42$$

The lower value for Market 1 indicates that it is more competitive than Market 2 with no dominant organization. A more competitive or concentrated market typically indicates potential challenges for growing profitable volume and emphasizes the need to define a competitive differentiation.

Achieving a Competitive Differentiation: What Sets Your Organization Apart?

A **competitive differentiation** is what sets an organization apart from others in the market. Leaders must continuously and consistently define and pursue strategies to achieve and sustain a competitive differentiation from rival organizations in the market.

According to Porter,[4] an organization can be differentiated from its competitors by being unique at something that is valued by its customers. The three types of competitive differentiation shown in Box 8.8 are quality, service, and cost.

BOX 8.8

TYPES OF COMPETITIVE DIFFERENTIATION
1. Quality
2. Service
3. Cost

Quality Differentiation

Clinical quality is achieving an intended outcome without causing undue harm to the patient. Broadly this translates to improving morbidity and mortality for a specified medical condition. While most healthcare provider organizations state that high quality care is their primary goal, improving patients' health status depends upon many variables within and outside the control of the healthcare provider organization. For example, clinicians' strict adherence to evidence-based medical safety and clinical protocols such as proper hand hygiene prevents the spread of hospital-acquired infection.

This is a significant challenge to the physicians' Hippocratic Oath of "first, do no harm"[5] given that preventable medical errors are attributed to an estimated 44,000 to 98,000 avoidable deaths in the United States each year.[6]

Patients also have an important role in their health outcomes through compliance with the treatment plan, including taking the prescribed medications, following a healthy diet, and exercising regularly. Most patients without clinical backgrounds use proxies to evaluate the "quality" of their experience with the healthcare provider organization, such as the convenience of accessing services, cleanliness of the facilities, and most important the friendliness and caring attitude of the providers and staff.

Service Differentiation

Providing exceptional service is *the* key differentiator in creating and sustaining a competitive advantage to growing profitable volume and market share. Unrivaled service excellence is a cultural imperative to achieving the organization's growth goals. Beyond offering convenient access to services, providers and staff whom patients and family members encounter throughout their visit make a memorable impression, favorably or unfavorably, that will largely determine if the patient and family members will return and refer others. Every encounter from housekeepers to nurses is an opportunity to strengthen the organization's brand and potential for word-of-mouth referrals to increase business—or not.

Consider an especially bad experience eating out at a restaurant. Did you return? Did you tell others about your experience? According to research,[7] most dissatisfied customers won't complain and might defect to a competitor. However, if employees are empowered to identify and quickly resolve their complaint they are likely to return and create new business. This approach is known as **service recovery**, actions taken typically as part of a formal program to convert customer issues to increase loyal customers. For example, a front desk receptionist acknowledging a patient is upset after waiting 30 minutes past her scheduled appointment offers her an apology and voucher for a free meal in the cafeteria for the inconvenience. The cost of a meal can make all the difference to retain existing patients and attract new patients, understanding that it costs five to six times as much to get a new first time customer as it does to keep a current one. The impact of customer service, positive or negative, outlined in Box 8.9 is the same for any service-driven industry.

Cost Differentiation

With the movement and increasing momentum to value-based care and reimbursement, being the low-cost provider can support achieving a competitive advantage in the market to grow profitable volume and market share. This is especially important given the growing interest in pricing transparency to disclose how much patients and other payers pay for care. Consistently providing services at a relatively lower cost (and higher quality) than competitors is especially attractive to patients and other payers given increasingly high consumer

---

BOX 8.9

IMPACT OF CUSTOMER SERVICE

- One in 25 customers will complain.
- Dissatisfied customers will tell nine to 15 people.
- Thirteen percent will tell 20 or more people.
- If their problem is resolved, 56% to 70% of customers who complain will return.
- Ninety-six percent of customers will return and tell four to six people about their positive experience if they believe the organization acted quickly and to their satisfaction.

---

out-of-pocket expense. What's more, managed care organizations and large employers are negotiating aggressively with healthcare provider organizations to deliver better value to their members or employees. Among the actions that leaders can take to reduce expense to achieve cost differentiation are improving throughput and capacity to lower unit of service costs and negotiating lower input costs with vendors.

STEP 4. Define the Value Proposition

The next step in the growth process is to define the business enterprise's value proposition. A **value proposition** is an innovation, service, or feature that make a product or service attractive to customers. It is the promise of value that will be delivered by the organization to meet or exceed customers' expectations. Leaders can develop an effective value proposition through establishing a clear understanding of their customers' needs and expectations. A value proposition can apply to the entire healthcare provider organization or to a specific business enterprise. An organization's value proposition should describe how its services address common challenges experienced by patients. For example "quality healthcare made easier" or "partners in your well-being" are value propositions that address the frustrations patients often encounter accessing care or lack of communication with their care team. A value proposition paints a clear picture of what the business enterprise brand can offer its customers compared to its competitors.

While the value proposition should always be defined from the customers' perspective and based solely on their expectation, services are unfortunately often built from the inside out or from the perspective of what's convenient for providers and staff rather than what's easier for patients. For example, the entire clinic closing during lunch when patients are completing errands, such as making an appointment to see their provider, is an inside-out approach and counterintuitive to growing volume. A common derivation of the inside out approach is "build it and they will come" whereby leaders make broad assumptions of what their customers want or need that may not be accurate. Writing an effective value proposition that captures the essence of what competitively differentiates the healthcare provider organization from others in the market should address the three components listed in Box 8.10: capability, impact, and proof.[8]

BOX 8.10

VALUE PROPOSITION COMPONENTS
1. Capability
2. Impact
3. Proof

Capability addresses why the business enterprise is the best or most able to provide the service, such as the qualifications of its providers or its adoption of leading-edge technology. *Impact* is how the service will have a positive impact on customers, such as ease of access, unparalleled customer service, or adherence to strict patient safety and clinical quality standards. Impact explains how the healthcare provider organization can fulfill a customer's needs or solve a problem better than competing organizations. *Proof* is providing evidence of how the service will have a positive impact on customers, such as through sharing objective consumer reports and recognition. Proof supports an organization's claims of its capability and impact. For example, an organization's value proposition "unparalleled commitment to performance excellence" is supported by announcing it won the prestigious Malcolm Baldrige Award.

STEP 5. Develop and Implement the Growth Plan

The final step in growing incremental volume and market share is putting together all of the previously developed components of the blueprint into a well-defined plan with actionable and measurable objectives for leadership accountability. Box 8.11 presents the steps for developing and implementing an effective growth plan beginning with sizing and prioritizing the potential opportunities, introducing standards for access and service, identifying and engaging key referral sources, and promoting accountability for ensuring the value proposition is upheld.

BOX 8.11

DEVELOPING AND IMPLEMENTING THE GROWTH PLAN
STEP 5.1. Identify and prioritize growth opportunities.
STEP 5.2. Define access and service standards.
STEP 5.3. Identify and engage referral sources.
STEP 5.4. Deliver on the promise.

STEP 5.1. Identify and Prioritize Growth Opportunities

Taking an objective, quantifiable, and data-driven approach to identify and validate growth opportunities removes the potential inherent bias of stakeholder interests that may not be fully aligned with the organization's strategic goals. The bubble graph presented in Figure 8.3 shows the projected average annual growth rate in the market on the horizontal axis and the contribution margin on the vertical axis. The size of the bubble relates the growth potential to enable focusing on the right services based on the projected contribution margin and the average annual growth rate. Recall from Chapter 4 that the contribution margin is calculated by subtracting only the variable costs from

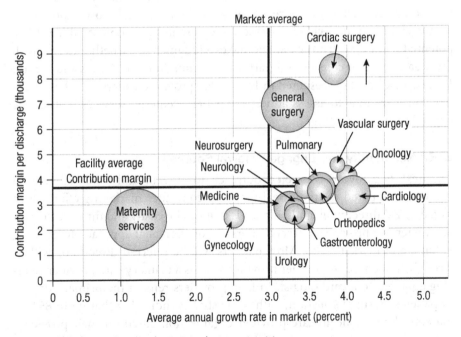

FIGURE 8.3 Assessing market growth opportunities.
Source: Reproduced with permission from Gee EP. *Service Line Success: Eight Essential Rules.* Health Administration Press; 2004.

operating revenue. Average annual growth rate can be determined by using the method for estimating total potential volume addressed previously. This approach also promotes prioritizing and allocating scarce resources to the growth initiatives that have the highest potential return on investment (ROI). For example, maternity services is a growth opportunity based on the size of the bubble, however its position in the lower left quadrant shows relatively lower profitability and annual growth rate compared to general and cardiac surgery in the upper right quadrant of the graph.

STEP 5.2. Define Access and Service Standards

As previously discussed the organization's ability to deliver easily accessible and patient-centered services is the key to achieving a competitive differentiation. Patient loyalty and return business is largely based on the quality of the overall experience, especially access and service, and not solely on the quality of the clinical care delivered. High touch service and access are patients' proxy for quality. Leaders must therefore strive to develop, implement, and monitor standards for ensuring easily accessible, highly personalized service. Every interaction a patient has with the healthcare provider organization potentially creates an opportunity to influence their returning and creating new business—or not.

Every encounter the patient has from the telephone demeanor of a scheduler, to eye contact with the receptionist at the front desk, to the provider's compassion and undivided attention—represents a "moment of truth," a potential point at which the patient makes a judgment on whether to stay with the organization or consider migrating to a competitor. The Access and Service Excellence Checklist presented in Exhibit 8.3 provides leaders with best practice considerations to assess and create patient-centered services that can be applied to any care setting.

STEP 5.3. Identify and Engage Referral Sources

The next step involves targeted outreach to current and potential referral sources. Compared to traditional direct-to-consumer marketing efforts such as radio, TV, direct mail, and billboards that can be costly and difficult to track ROI, referring provider outreach offers a more personal approach to growing volume and market share. Most patients will be referred directly or will be strongly influenced by another provider such as a primary care provider referring a patient to a cardiologist. In fact, providers remain the primary drivers of patients' hospital selection, with some studies indicating that up to 85% of patients choose a healthcare provider organization based on their provider's recommendation.[1,9] The process of identifying all referral sources, both current and potential, can be structured into three distinct phases listed in Figure 8.4.

EXHIBIT 8.3

ACCESS AND SERVICE EXCELLENCE CHECKLIST

ACCESS AND SERVICE EXCELLENCE	OFFERED	
	YES	NO
Access		
Appointment availability: Routine ≤1 week		
Appointment availability: Urgent same day		
Same-day/walk-in appointments		
Lunchtime appointments		
Evening hours offered		
Weekend hours offered		
Follow-up appointment made before patient leaves		
Online patient portal for scheduling and communication		
Patients in waiting room ≤15 minutes		
Emergency department wait time (time to physician ≤30 minutes)		
Service		
Reminder call, text, or email to patients (based on their communication preference) within 48 hours of appointment		
Follow-up calls to no-show or cancelled appointment patients (service recovery)		
On-site diagnostic testing		
Call patients with test results within 3 days		
Protocols and training for staff phone etiquette		
Staff empowered to resolve patient problems (service recovery program)		
Free or subsidized parking		
Adequate signage and wayfinding		
Facilities clean and updated		
Patients referred to as Mr. or Ms.		
Cloth gowns versus paper gowns		
Weight scale not in publicly visible area		
Public health guidelines followed (masks, social distancing)		
Patient privacy safeguarded at all times (HIPAA)		
Access and service performance measures collected and reviewed weekly with key stakeholders, action plans addressing opportunities developed, implemented, and monitored		

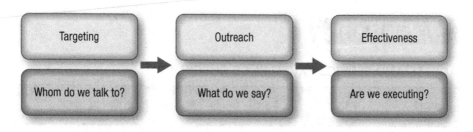

FIGURE 8.4 Phases of referral outreach.

Targeting

The first phase of referral outreach is identifying which providers are critical to the organization's strategic and financial growth goals. Referring providers can be segmented into four categories according to their affiliation with and affinity to the healthcare provider organization: loyal, splitter, loosely affiliated, and not affiliated according to their referral volume. Current and potential referring providers can further be stratified by clinical service line and profitability. Table 8.7 shows the recommended amount of time and outreach effort that should be spent on each group based on a typical return in investment in incremental volume.

Loyal providers refer 80% or more of their total volume to the business enterprise. Employed providers should but do not always fall in to this category. Referral volume from loyal, especially employed, providers should be closely tracked to make sure the organization is preventing leakage to competitors and retaining as much volume within the system as possible. Acceptable exceptions to patient volume outmigration include if a service is not available, the patient's insurance is not accepted, or strong patient preference. Techniques to discuss referral leakage with referring providers will be addressed later in the chapter. Referring providers who split their referrals among two or more different healthcare provider organizations represent a significant opportunity

TABLE 8.7 Referring Provider Categories and Suggested Allocation of Effort

REFERRING PROVIDER CATEGORY	PERCENT OF TOTAL REFERRAL VOLUME	OUTREACH EFFORT/ RESOURCE ALLOCATION
Loyal (employed or contracted)	80%–100%	20%
Splitter	20%–80%	60%
Loosely affiliated	1%–20%	10%
No relationship (not on medical staff)	0%	10%

for increasing volume and market share. Providers already exhibiting a preference for referring at least half to three quarters of their current business can further be stratified and prioritized to identify potential "high-yield" provider opportunities to increase referrals.

Targeting the right splitters provides an opportunity to maximize the return on outreach efforts that increase profitable volume and market share. Loosely affiliated providers typically only refer or admit less than 20% of their patients when absolutely required typically due to call obligations, patient or referring provider preference, or insurance network limitations. Lastly, a modest amount of time should be allocated to providers who are in the market but not currently on the healthcare provider organization's medical staff, though typically with a low ROI and subject to legal anti-competitive constraints.

Outreach

A deliberate, well-defined value proposition should be developed similar to that of the broader healthcare provider organization. The value proposition for the business enterprise should be tailored to the specific needs and expectations of the referring provider group rather than taking a "one size fits all" approach. For example, Exhibit 8.4 presents a sample value proposition for surgeons based on their need for high quality, patient safety, efficiency, and service.

Growing incremental volume relies on reaching out to current and potential referring providers and simply asking for their business.

EXHIBIT 8.4

REFERRING PROVIDER VALUE PROPOSITION (SURGEON EXAMPLE)

Quality and safety	• Nurse-to-patient ratios higher than national average and local hospitals to ensure safer, more personalized care
Efficiency	• Easily accessible operating rooms with simple and flexible "open" scheduling • Increased patient throughput from highly-trained specialized staff to provide faster operating room turnaround times • Streamlined workflow by seamlessly providing both inpatient and outpatient services within the same operating room setting • Minimized operating room time through leading-edge technology
Service	• Patient-centered care with the convenience of comprehensive services under one roof (therapy, imaging, lab, pharmacy) • Leadership responsive to physician needs allowing them to focus on patient care • Access imaging reports and studies from anywhere (home, office, clinic) • Streamlined patient registration process to avoid delays

The messaging to the targeted referring providers must be clear, concise, consistent, and centered around their and their patients' needs. This is known as a "seller-based" versus a "buyer-based" outreach. An effective outreach approach is asking current and potential referral sources:

"*What can we do to earn more of your business*" or "*What can we do to make the experience better for you and your patients?*"

Leaders must be responsive and continuously follow-up with referring providers to act on the feedback and opportunities they present for earning more of their business. Doing so strengthens the necessary trust for a productive and sustainable relationship.

Effectiveness

The effectiveness of the organization's outreach effort is apparent in tracking referrals, as shown in Exhibit 8.5, typically on a monthly basis. High-value current and potential referral sources can be prioritized to allocate the proportionate effort and outreach resources based on the potential ROI. Referring provider data can be obtained from a number of sources including internal utilization reports, provider practice databases, vendor intelligence and market analyses, and state databases.

EXHIBIT 8.5

REFERRING PROVIDER TRACKING EXAMPLE

REFERRING PROVIDER	SPECIALTY	BUSINESS ENTERPRISE	COMPETITOR 1	COMPETITOR 2	TOTAL
Adams, J.	Internal Medicine	37%	12%	51%	100%
Evans, G.	Internal Medicine	15%	51%	34%	100%
Moore, T.	Cardiology	45%	55%	0%	100%
Smith, M.	Family Practice	31%	22%	47%	100%
Williams, L.	Orthopedic Surgery	17%	34%	49%	100%

Measuring Impact of Incremental Referral Volume

Assessing the ROI of various volume and market share growth initiatives including increased referring provider activity is important for leaders to evaluate and prioritize opportunities. Calculating ROI for a specific growth initiative can be accomplished by identifying the change in volume and revenue assumed to be the result of the initiative, shown by the formula in Box 8.12.

BOX 8.12

CALCULATING INCREMENTAL REFERRING PROVIDER REVENUE

Incremental referring provider revenue = (Total volume after initiative × Average net revenue per encounter) − (Baseline referral volume × Average revenue per encounter)

For example, outreach efforts to increase outpatient diagnostic imaging referrals from a busy family practice clinic of 6 providers can be measured and monitored. The practice's average monthly referral volume was 10 MRI and 5 CT scans per month in the previous 12 months. Upon working with the practice administrator to make the test ordering process easier through a computerized provider order entry system, the clinic increases the number of monthly MRI and CT scans to 15 and 10, respectively, over the next 6 months. The average net revenue for an MRI is $350 and $500 for a CT scan. The incremental revenue can be calculated follows:

$$\text{Incremental referring provider revenue} = (15 \text{ MRI} \times \$350) + (10 \text{ CT } \$500) -$$
$$(10 \text{ MRI} \times \$350) + (5 \text{ CT } \$500)$$
$$= \$10,250 - \$6,000$$
$$= \$4,250 \text{ incremental revenue}$$

STEP 5.4. Deliver on the Promise

Patients usually have a choice of healthcare provider organizations from which they can seek care. Providing comparatively better customer service usually correlates to higher volume compared to organizations that do not. Leaders have significant influence over access to care and the environment in which patients receive care, specifically how patients and their families are treated, made to feel comfortable, and respected. Referring and attending providers are also "customers" who can elect to treat or refer their patients where they believe they'll get the best outcome, service, and overall experience.

Beyond all of the planning, assessing, and prioritizing of organizational resources and effort, the most critical aspect of effective growth planning is delivering on the promise of value—meeting or exceeding customers' needs and expectations. This is achieved through leaders' continuous measuring, monitoring, and managing all of the actions and events to provide unparalleled service. Using available customer service metrics and dashboards to evaluate opportunities for improvement is paramount to achieving the organization's financial goals.

REGIONAL HEALTH SYSTEM CASE EXAMPLE: GROWTH TASK FORCE INITIATIVES

After identifying the opportunities to reduce unnecessary operating expense detailed in Chapters 6 and 7 from the financial condition analysis presented in Chapter 4, the Director of Surgical Services next turned her focus to growing profitable volume and market share as part of a system-wide task force to increase operating revenue. The task force was comprised of multidisciplinary expertise including strategic planning, business development, clinical service lines, operations, and finance. Among the growth initiatives presented by the task force to Regional Health System's (RHS) senior leadership are a "Welcome to Medicare" initiative, Lobby Screening Program, and Referring Provider Liaison Program.

"Welcome to Medicare" Initiative

The baby boom generation born after World War II between 1946 and 1964 is aging into Medicare health insurance eligibility at the rate of about 10,000 Americans per day.[9,10] The "silver tsunami" presents a significant opportunity to capture more business from this population, typically the largest payer by volume and revenue for most healthcare provider organizations. Transitioning to Medicare can be a stressful and confusing time as baby boomers try to navigate their new eligibility and what services are covered.

Assessing the demographics of the RHS's PSA and SSA, the growth task force identified several trends. First, based on census data, the total population was expected to increase by 12% in its PSA and 9% in its SSA over the next 10 years as shown in Table 8.8. Further analysis identified that nearly two-thirds of the expected growth was from people aged 65 and older due to the increasing retirement popularity of the region. Regional disease prevalence data indicated that this population was at significantly higher risk for the common chronic diseases including heart disease, diabetes, and cancer.

RHS plans to mail "Welcome to Medicare" packets to all residents in its service areas 6 months before they turn 65 to notify them of the free benefits to which they are entitled, such as a visit with a physician to review their medical and social history, and provide education and counseling about covered

TABLE 8.8 Regional Health System's Service Area Population and Demographics (20X3–20Y3)

SERVICE AREA	CURRENT POPULATION 20X3	PROJECTED POPULATION 20Y3	VARIANCE	VARIANCE PERCENT
Primary service area (PSA)	157,683	179,605	21,922	12.2%
>65 years	28,383	42,632.24	14,249	33.4%
Secondary service area (SSA)	126,146	137,499	11,353	8.3%
>65 years	27,752	35,132	7,380	21.0%

preventive services and screening tests. RHS will include in the packet helpful information about how to access the services, such as the direct access number for scheduling the preventive visit and the range and location of comprehensive services it provides.

RHS projects that the initiative will result in scheduling 15 new Medicare beneficiary visits per month that would have not otherwise established a relationship with the system. The average annual net revenue per Medicare patient is $5,700 including all diagnostic testing, outpatient visits, and acute inpatient care. The incremental overhead cost to support the program, including additional staffing and supplies, is estimated to be 40% of the projected revenue. The expected annual cost to purchase the mailing list, mail the packets, and administer the program is $30,000. The projected downstream revenue from all care resulting from this market segment is $585,600 (see Table 8.9).

TABLE 8.9 Regional Health System's Projected "Welcome to Medicare" Revenue (20X3)

Volume	
Beneficiaries establishing new patient relationship	180
Revenue (acute care, outpatient, and ancillary services)	
Total revenue	$1,026,000
Expense	
Overhead (staff, clinic space, supplies)	$410,400
Program administration (mailing campaign)	$30,000
Total expense	$440,400
Net income	$585,600

"Lobby Screening" Initiative

A member of the RHS task force and cardiovascular service line administrator shared an anecdotal story from one of the employed interventional cardiologists who remarked how interested her patients' family members were and began including them in the discussion (with the patients' permission) about the diagnosis, proposed treatment, and preventive measures for the sake of the patients' family members. She noted that the family members likely had the same genetic and lifestyle risk factors that cause heart disease, which can often go undetected until a heart attack or stroke occurs. Wanting to support increasing prevention and diagnosis of heart disease, the RHS Heart Clinic leadership decided to pilot a screening program in the organization's lobby augmenting part-time staffing with nursing students from the local college and also volunteers.

The Lobby Screening Initiative promotes community goodwill, strengthens provider relations, and creates downstream revenue by offering free "point of service" health screenings to visitors who are given their results and offered prevention education by a licensed vocational nurse. The screening includes body composition, blood pressure, glucose, cholesterol, nutrition assessment, heart attack/stroke risk, peripheral arterial disease (PAD) risk, and sleep apnea risk. "At-risk" visitors whose results fall outside the normal or recommend ranges are encouraged to follow-up with their primary care provider or are referred to an RHS PCP if they don't have one and an appropriate specialist.

The projected number of screenings that can be conducted per week over 50 weeks is 100 or 5,000 per year. An estimated 25% of the visitors screened are projected to be identified as "high risk" requiring follow-up diagnostic testing. Approximately 15% of patients who have a diagnostic test will require a procedure. Based on internal financial data the average net revenue per outpatient diagnostic study is $350 and the average net revenue per procedure is $7,500. Part-time labor expense to oversee and staff the program, test kits, and marketing materials will cost more than $40,000 per year. The projected annual ROI for the program is $421,550 (see Table 8.10).

Provider Liaison Program

Based on feedback from RHS's referring providers on opportunities to improve access and service to support patient safety and clinical quality initiatives, the RHS growth task force recommended developing a provider liaison program. Without dedicating efforts to secure loyalty, healthcare provider organizations risk losing volume to competitor facilities. Liaisons serve to strengthen the relationship with providers to improve quality and increase referrals. Unlike traditional marketing channels the provider liaison program

TABLE 8.10 **Regional Health System's Projected Lobby Screening Revenue (20X3)**

Volume	
Health screenings	5,000
High risk visitors	1,250
Follow-up diagnostic testing (stress, echo, CT)	313
Procedure (cardiac catheterization)	47
Revenue	
Diagnostic tests	$109,550
Procedures	$352,500
Total revenue	$462,050
Expense	
Labor (part-time LVN)	$28,500
Supplies and marketing	$12,000
Total expense	$40,500
Net income	$421,550

entails more direct, consultative sales through repetitive, face-to-face, and relationship-driven contact. By instituting this dual service and sales approach, provider liaisons are able to bolster referring provider satisfaction and loyalty.

The ultimate goal of the provider liaison program is relationship management to expand the referring provider base and in turn increase volume and market share. From a purely service perspective, the provider liaison may also provide referring providers with information on new services and procedures; serve as a personal contact for the referring provider to address questions, concerns or feedback; and facilitate access to a dedicated consultation and referral program. While the provider liaison program should be approached as a sales program from an internal strategy perspective, it should not be marketed as such to referring providers. Rather, the provider liaison should adopt a dual customer service and marketing approach, as customized provider attention is more likely to result in increased volumes.

While an important goal of the provider liaison program is to grow patient volume, leaders should be mindful not to sacrifice long-term provider relationships for short-term business gains. RHS plans to pilot the liaison program by hiring three representatives. (See Appendix H for a sample job description.) RHS projects that the initiative will result in increasing referring provider volume by 14% in the first year of the program net of operating expenses and $165,000 in net income.

The total projected RHS annual incremental net revenue for FY 20X3 from implementing the task force's recommended growth initiatives is $1,172,150, summarized in Table 8.11.

TABLE 8.11 **Growth Initiatives Projected Financial Impact**

GROWTH INITIATIVE	FINANCIAL IMPACT
1. "Welcome to Medicare"	$585,600
2. Lobby Screening	$421,550
3. Referring Provider Liaison	$165,000
Total projected annual revenue increase	$1,172,150

SUMMARY

Growing profitable volume and market share is essential to support the organization's mission and achieve its strategic and financial goals. Leaders are responsible for developing, implementing, and continuously monitoring a deliberate and comprehensive growth plan that includes assessing market demographics, competitors, and referring providers. Simultaneously identifying and satisfying the needs and expectations of referring providers and their patients support the goal of growing profitable volume and market share.

CALLS TO ACTION

Leaders should:

- Monitor population demographics and population health data to evaluate and deliver services on patients' needs and service expectations.

- Evaluate market rivals to identify opportunities for competitive differentiation.

- Engage current and referring providers to ask how more of their business can be earned.

References

1. Sachs/Scarborough HealthPlus Study. Market Study. 1999.
2. Centers for Disease Control and Prevention. Prevalence of heart disease—United States, 2005. *MMWR*. 2007;56(6):113-118.
3. Terwiesch C, Diwas KC, Kahn JM. Working with capacity limitations: operations management in critical care. *Crit Care*. 2011;15(4):308.
4. Porter ME. *Competitive Advantage: Creating and Sustaining Superior Performance*. The Free Press; 1985.
5. Edelstein L. *The Hippocratic Oath: Text, Translation and Interpretation*. The Johns Hopkins Press; 1943.
6. Institute of Medicine. *To Err is Human: Building a Safer Health System*. The National Academies Press; 2000.

7. White House Office of Consumer Affairs. 2004.
8. Rackham N, DeVincentis JR. *Rethinking the Sales Force: Redefining Selling to Create and Capture Customer Value*. McGraw-Hill; 1999.
9. Gee EP. *Service Line Success: Eight Essential Rules*. Health Administration Press; 2004.
10. U.S. Census Bureau, 2010 Census. www.census.gov

PART V

MONITORING

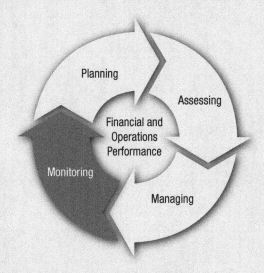

INTRODUCTION TO MONITORING

A critical role and responsibility of leaders is making effective decisions about how to allocate scarce resources to support the organization's mission and to achieve its strategic goals. As there is often a disconnect between the planned goal and the actual results, continuous monitoring is required. The results from the actions taken in the Managing Phase should be compared to internal and external benchmarks, such as a balanced scorecard or performance measurement dashboard, to enable leaders' taking the necessary corrective actions. Leaders should strive to anticipate any variance to the planned result or performance measurement target through deliberate contingency plans rather than react to unexpected changes.

CHAPTER 9

MAKING THE BUSINESS CASE FOR QUALITY

LEARNING OBJECTIVES

- Adopt a deliberate business case approach to calculate and prioritize return on investment (ROI) for performance improvement initiatives.
- Calculate the cost of waste (COW) of poor quality.
- Monetize quality improvement initiatives using one or more proven techniques to estimate financial impact.
- Link quality and cost using an integrated performance improvement scorecard.
- Use rapid cycle testing to overcome risk aversion and fiscal austerity.

TOOLS AND TECHNIQUES

- Business case analysis
- Monetizing quality
- Problem and goal statement writing
- Rapid cycle testing

KEY TERMS AND CONCEPTS

Business case	Cycle time
Waste	Cost-to-charge ratio (CCR)
Process of care	Opportunity cost
Mode of care	Cost avoidance
Cost of waste	Return on investment (ROI)
Process map	

INTRODUCTION

Healthcare leaders are under growing pressure to continuously improve quality while simultaneously eliminating waste and cutting unnecessary costs. The dual challenge is driven largely by changing reimbursement models. In addition to government value-based care and pay-for-performance programs, private health insurance organizations and large employers are increasingly seeking exclusive partnerships through narrow networks with healthcare provider organizations that consistently demonstrate value: The highest quality at the lowest cost. However, leaders often struggle with aligning their mission and strategic goals with the business case for them. Connecting quality improvement to the anticipated financial impact is challenging due to data constraints, a language barrier between providers and administrators, limited financial management acumen, and lack of provider alignment. Surviving in a value-based care environment requires making a sound business case.

A **business case** is an effective evaluative tool used to project the financial impact and feasibility of a quality improvement initiative. The goal of a business case is to support and inform leadership decision-making to improve organizational performance improvement by identifying and prioritizing opportunities that have the greatest impact. A sound business case provides a systematic method for allocating scarce resources based on the organization's mission and strategic goals. The business case explores the potential cost-benefit of various scenarios for a project through exploring "what if" scenarios through a sensitivity analysis, presented in Chapter 10.

KEY CRITERIA FOR AN EFFECTIVE BUSINESS CASE

A good business case achieves the criteria presented in Box 9.1. It should include and weigh all possible variables that could affect the financial feasibility of the project, both quantitative and qualitative. A well-designed business case should also be simple to understand and easy to explain to key stakeholders for getting their feedback and buy-in to the proposed initiative. A sound business case should take a conservative approach for estimating the financial impact of the project. It should establish realistic targets and expectations for achieving them, including the potential for unforeseen complications and risks such as a new competitor entering the market, increased cost of labor and supplies due to shortages, or internal leadership turbulence causing turnover. Last and most important, an effective business case should be developed with a focus on achieving measurable results through implementation. Beyond being a useful planning tool, a good business case should establish a clear pathway to follow through and implement the proposed opportunity to improve organizational performance.

BOX 9.1

KEY CRITERIA FOR AN EFFECTIVE BUSINESS CASE
1. Comprehensive
2. Simple
3. Conservative
4. Actionable

APPLYING THE BUSINESS CASE APPROACH

The business case is traditionally used and often required by investors, financial institutions, and governing boards for large capital projects such as a new building, equipment, joint venture, or merger or acquisition. The business case is less commonly used for other applications, including developing or expanding a clinical service or service line, hiring a new provider, and evaluating clinical efficacy and cost-effectiveness of two or more potential options. The business case helps to identify the potential financial risk or exposure of a proposed project. Risk management and mitigation methods are addressed in Chapter 10.

When considering potential business case applications leaders will find it useful to first frame the financial impact of a future project by identifying the specific problem and the goal they want to accomplish. Often leaders rush to a solution before completely understanding the problem they are trying to resolve. A well-written **problem statement** should create a compelling case that clearly identifies the central issue including who is affected by the current situation and how. It should also have a "call to action"; that is, why the problem needs to be addressed and by when. Leaders should resist the common temptation of embedding a solution into the problem statement at the risk of eliminating other potential solutions. Identifying the goal for an initiative becomes easier once the problem is clearly defined. An effective **goal statement** should include all of the elements presented in Box 9.2 including the specific process to be improved, quantifiable performance measurement, and when the goal should be achieved. Clearly defining the specific problem and goal is important to engage and inform key stakeholders.

> ## BOX 9.2
>
> DEVELOPING A *SMART* GOAL
> **S**pecific
> **M**easurable
> **A**chievable
> **R**elevant
> **T**ime-oriented

CHALLENGES TO CREATING THE BUSINESS CASE

There are several challenges to creating an effective business case, shown in Box 9.3, including data limitations, financial language barriers, lacking financial acumen in the business of health, and weak alignment with providers.

> ## BOX 9.3
>
> CHALLENGES TO CREATING AN EFFECTIVE BUSINESS CASE
> 1. Data limitations
> 2. Financial language barrier
> 3. Financial acumen
> 4. Alignment with providers

Many healthcare provider organizations have difficulty providing timely, accurate, and actionable data to support effective leadership decision-making. While considerable data is collected from every facet of the organization, it is challenging for leaders to translate it into useful information and insights to support performance improvement efforts. What's more, there is rarely a seamless interface and integration between the often disparate clinical, operations and financial data collection systems and reports.

Healthcare provider organizations have invested heavily in clinical information systems such as electronic health records to improve patient quality and safety often at the expense of developing the necessary business intelligence and financial management systems to run the enterprise. Organizations are further challenged with providing valid and reliable data. Lacking data collection processes leads to poor end results also known as "garbage in, garbage out."

Beyond these common data constraints leaders are sometimes reluctant to share financial information with key stakeholders, including providers, largely out of concern about its accuracy and their inability to interpret the information, creating a language barrier between clinical and financial leaders.

Clinical leaders also have difficulty translating patient safety and quality improvement goals into bottom line justification for the resources required to achieve them. The lack of understanding and inability to translate clinical needs into a business case is a common source of tension among clinicians. At the same time, administrative leaders struggle with justifying the need to support additional and often unbudgeted expenses to support their patient care mission. The language gap is further exacerbated by a general lack of financial acumen in the business of health among many leaders. Critical financial decisions that affect the organization are often made in a vacuum due to limited discussion and lacking integration of clinical efficacy and financial efficiency.

Both clinical and administrative leaders are often limited in their technical skill, current knowledge, and confident ability to use basic financial management and operations know-how to drive meaningful performance improvement throughout their organizations. This is especially true for clinicians, despite their significant influence on the bottom line. Moreover, most graduate-level higher education programs in healthcare or business administration focus too much on theory and too little on practical application.

A final hindrance to leaders' making an effective business case is the lack of alignment with their medical staff contributing to thinning operating margins and poor quality outcomes.[1,2] Alignment is the degree of unity of purpose and existence of mutually beneficial goals between providers and the business enterprise. According to management guru Peter Drucker, "You can't manage what you can't measure." Defining and measuring alignment are imposing challenges that leaders can overcome using the research-based Alignment Survey provided in Appendix I addressing the critical domains in Table 9.1.

Leaders can use the objective and unbiased survey results to validate their current strategic alignment direction, benchmark alignment strategy with evidence-based best practices, and establish a baseline for measuring the effectiveness of future initiatives. Leaders aiming to overcome the barriers to alignment are likely to be more effective by educating providers in the process of building a sound business case to better integrate quality improvement and financial goals.

FIVE-STEP PROCESS FOR MAKING AN EFFECTIVE BUSINESS CASE

An effective approach for making a sound business case involves five simple and sequential steps, listed in Box 9.4. After identifying the specific opportunity

TABLE 9.1 **Alignment Survey Domains and Definitions**

DOMAIN	DEFINITION
Rule Making	Instituting evidence-based best practices through required use of organization-provided tools and processes
Communicating Performance	Giving providers accurate, timely, and actionable data
Supported Change	Offering providers "how to" instruction, training and education, and ongoing coaching and mentoring to achieve best practices
Governance and Leadership	Installing and cultivating formal physician leaders throughout all levels of the organization to set and achieve strategic goals
Structural Model	Creating formal organization-sponsored relationships with physicians enabling participating in risk/reward models
Risk and Reward	Offering "skin in the game" pay-for-performance bonuses and/or risk-based penalties based on achieving specified physician-driven goals
Sociological-Cultural	Creating organizational culture fostering trust, collaboration, intrinsic motivation to achieve the organization's goals

for improvement such as an unsafe, ineffective, or inefficient process, leaders must calculate the current or projected cost of waste associated with it. Next, the anticipated cost of the proposed intervention must be determined. Based on a reasonable and conservative forecast the estimated impact of the quality improvement initiative must be monetized, such as how much the project will save over a specified period of time. Lastly, the cost of waste must be compared to the projected return expected from the proposed initiative.

BOX 9.4

FIVE STEPS FOR MAKING AN EFFECTIVE BUSINESS CASE
STEP 1. Identify the performance improvement opportunity.
STEP 2. Calculate the cost of waste.
STEP 3. Determine the cost of the proposed solution.
STEP 4. Project the anticipated financial impact.
STEP 5. Calculate the return on investment.

STEP 1. Identify the Performance Improvement Opportunity

There is no shortage of opportunities to reduce waste and inefficiency in healthcare. Industry experts estimate the amount of waste causing significant

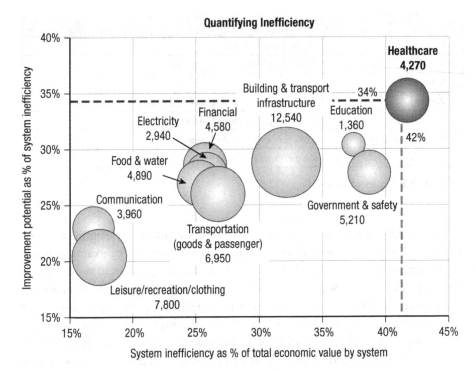

FIGURE 9.1 Comparative industry waste.
Source: IBM. Redefining value and success in healthcare: charting the path to the future. Whitepaper: IBM Healthcare and Life Sciences Thought Leadership. January 2012.

unnecessary cost is between one quarter and one third[3] and perhaps even higher relative to other industries as shown in Figure 9.1.

Waste is anything that does not support improving health outcomes. The underlying causes of waste include failure of care delivery, failure of care coordination, overtreatment, excessive prices, administrative complexity, and fraud and abuse.[4,5] The greatest opportunities for reducing waste and unnecessary expense typically occur within complicated, multi-step processes that cross several departmental lines or functional areas where breakdowns and inefficiencies traditionally occur within silos. The common types of waste from the Lean manufacturing management philosophy primarily derived from the Toyota Production System can be applied to healthcare, shown in Figure 9.2.

There are two primary categories for considering potential performance improvement opportunities to reduce or eliminate waste: process of care and mode of care.

Process of care involves all of the functions and systems for delivering healthcare services.

CATEGORY OF WASTE	DEFINITION
1. Transportation	Moving stuff around
2. Inventory	Anything of value waiting in process
3. Motion	Excess movement
4. Waiting	Idle staff, equipment, capacity, the next step
5. Overproduction	Producing more than needed
6. Over-processing	Extra non-value-added steps
7. Defects	Waste, mistakes, pain

FIGURE 9.2 Types of waste.

Opportunities for cutting waste include streamlining, re-engineering, or leveraging technology to improve cumbersome processes. For example, offering an online registration and appointment scheduling system to reduce clinic labor and expense. **Mode of care** is all of the clinical settings in which patients are treated. Industry experts consistently identify unnecessary treatment or over-treatment as a significant contributor to the high and increasing cost of care.[6] Opportunities for reducing waste include eliminating non-value-added tests and treatment and delivering care in the most effective and conservative setting. Examples include non-critical patients treated in an intensive care unit who could safely be treated in a less acute and costly care setting.

STEP 2. Calculate the Cost of Waste

The next step in making an effective business case is to define and quantify the current cost of waste for the performance improvement opportunity identified in Step 1. The **cost of waste** or the cost of poor quality is the total measurable expense incurred by the business enterprise caused by clinically ineffective care and administratively inefficient processes. Identifying the cost of waste can be a very powerful motivator and catalyst for improving quality. Leaders may not understand the full scope or magnitude of implementing a performance improvement opportunity unless and until it is quantified into a dollar amount. Placing a dollar value on all quality improvement opportunities provides a common denominator to support comparing and prioritizing multiple and competing performance improvement initiatives. Estimating the cost of waste also helps translate patient safety and clinical care issues into the "language of finance" to which "classically-trained" healthcare leaders can relate.

Access to accurate and actionable financial data is a common rate-limiting factor in many healthcare provider organizations. Ninety percent of surveyed executives admitted they lacked a cost accounting system capable of providing the necessary financial data across the continuum of care.[7] In fact, according to the Healthcare Financial Management Association[8] most organizations claim that their current cost accounting system does not provide all of the information needed to support effective managerial decision-making. Nevertheless, since perfect data does not exist leaders should not be deterred from identifying the cost of waste.

Internal data provided from a cost accounting system *should* be the primary and most reliable source of accurate and actionable information to enable leaders' making timely and effective decisions. However, the dearth of accurate patient level cost data, especially when attempting to identify actual costs across multiple services or service lines, limits effective leadership decision-making. Leaders are therefore and rightfully reluctant to rely on cost data contained in financial reports. Using consistent and conservative measurement methods with reasonable assumptions can provide informed calculations with reliable estimates. Leaders shouldn't sacrifice "good enough" for "great" when taking the first important step to determine the cost of an ineffective or inefficient process. In lieu of an accounting system there are several methods that can be used to estimate the cost of waste shown in Box 9.5.

BOX 9.5

SOURCES FOR DETERMINING COST OF WASTE
- Cost accounting system
- Manual data collection
- Chart audit
- Cost-to-charge ratio
- White paper and scholarly research

Manual Data Collection

Capturing the cost of waste manually can be time-consuming and tedious, however it is a better alternative to doing nothing. Manually calculating the cost of waste typically involves aggregating pieces of disparate data from multiple systems. Lacking a cost accounting system should not prohibit developing a process for reasonably assessing the cost of waste even on a periodic basis. Recalling from Chapters 6 and 7 that labor and non-labor expense comprise the bulk of the total operating expense, estimating the cost of waste should focus on these two areas.

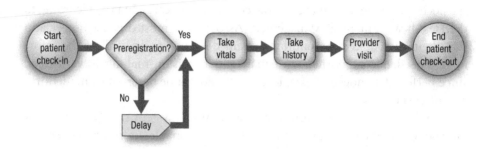

FIGURE 9.3 Process map example.

After identifying the unit of service such as an admission, outpatient visit, test, or procedure, determining the total productive hours spent by providers and staff can be achieved by combining two common process improvement techniques: process mapping and assessing average cycle time for each step in the process. Creating a **process map** or flow chart through direct and unbiased observation provides a detailed picture of all the steps and activities to assess problems or common areas of inefficiency such as decision points, waiting periods, bottlenecks, and tasks that must frequently be repeated. An example of a process map is shown in in Figure 9.3.

Once created the process map is used to identify the total amount of staff time spent during each step of the process or the total **cycle time**. Direct observation and collection of the same data for each process step over multiple iterations, ideally more than 30, will inform a defensible and reasonably accurate estimate of the average time to complete each step. For non-statisticians more than 30 data points is considered the minimum number of observations for a generally acceptable statistically significant sample size. Outlier data that would skew the results should be omitted from the analysis. As a general rule of thumb outliers are the highest and lowest values in the data set. An example of cycle times using the previous process map example is provided in Table 9.2.

Once the process map and cycle times are determined, the total cost of labor can be estimated by multiplying the total hourly labor rate by the average time spent per patient provided as shown in Table 9.3.

Chart Review

Reviewing clinical charts can provide important data that can be translated into useful financial information. Chart audits are traditionally performed to assess the completeness and the accuracy of patient data primarily for documentation and coding compliance to ensure the healthcare provider organization gets

TABLE 9.2 Determining Cycle Time

POSITION	AVERAGE TIME SPENT PER PATIENT: OUTPATIENT CLINIC (MINUTES)						TIME
	PROCESS STEPS						
	CHECK-IN	REGISTRATION	VITALS	HISTORY	VISIT	CHECKOUT	
Medical receptionist	6.0	4.3				3.4	13.7
Medical assistant			10.2				10.2
LVN				15.1			15.1
RN					19.2		19.2
Provider					17.5		17.5
Total time	6.0	4.3	10.2	15.1	36.7	3.4	75.7

TABLE 9.3 Determining Labor Expense

POSITION	HOURLY RATE	TIME SPENT PER PATIENT (MINUTES)	EXPENSE PER PATIENT
Medical receptionist	$14.18	13.7	$3.24
Medical assistant	$17.02	10.2	$2.89
LVN	$22.69	15.1	$5.71
RN	$28.37	19.2	$9.08
Provider	$85.10	17.5	$24.82
		Total labor expense per patient	$45.74

TABLE 9.4 Conducting a Chart Review

DRG195 Simple pneumonia & pleurisy w/o CC/MCC Modifier A04.72 Clostridium difficile not specified as recurrent	CDI not present on admission	CDI present on admission
	n = 30 charts	
Average length of stay	3.0 days	4.5 days

paid appropriately. Conducting a chart audit can also reveal useful information to estimate the cost of waste. For example, a chart audit can support identifying the adverse financial impact of treating a hospital-acquired condition, such as the common *Clostridium difficile* infection (CDI), by comparing a random sample of charts with and without the infection. As Table 9.4 shows, the same risk-adjusted diagnosis should be used to randomly draw at least 30 charts for each status.

Length of stay (LOS) or cost per patient day can be used as a reasonable proxy to determine total cost. Estimated cost per bed day should be available from the finance department. Otherwise cost per bed day according to the type of bed or cost per clinic visit can be calculated manually as previously discussed. Only direct and indirect expenses related to providing the service should be included in the total cost estimates. Recall from Chapter 2 that direct expense is tied to providing services, such as nursing care, and expendable medical supplies and indirect expense is for providing patient care support and services such as the clinical laboratory and housekeeping. Costs can also be approximated using the cost-to-charge ratio (CCR) method.

Cost-to-Charge Ratio

A common way to estimate cost is the CCR. Medicare uses CCRs to calculate outlier payments and DRG cost weighting. Leaders can apply CCR to approximate the cost of an admission, clinic visit, or other unit of service. The **CCR** is the ratio between a provider healthcare organization's expenses and what it

TABLE 9.5 **Calculating Cost Using Cost-to-Charge Ratio**

Number of hip replacements per month	30
Total charges (gross)	$900,000
Average charge per procedure	$30,000
Cost-to-charge ratio	40%
Estimated cost per procedure	$12,000

charges payers for services. The closer the ratio is to 1 the less difference there is between actual costs and charges. Multiplying the CCR by total charges provides an estimate of the cost of the service. The example in Table 9.5 shows the estimated cost for a hip replacement procedure using the CCR method. While the CCR is a simple approach that can be used to estimate total cost of a service it does not identify the cost of waste which must be estimated using best practice benchmarks. Benchmarking is addressed in Chapter 10.

White Paper or Scholarly Article

Published reports, either a white paper from a vendor or a research study from a scholarly journal, provide another potential source of cost information. However, many reports from vendors or consultants tend to be biased in favor of supporting the product or service they are selling. Mining valid and reliable financial information from journal articles is also a challenge since few clinical journal articles contain cost information. Also, the information may not be relevant by the time the study is published due to the significant lag. Nonetheless, both sources can be used as reasonable checks of the data identified in one of the previous other methods.

STEP 3. Determine the Cost of the Proposed Solution

Identifying the cost of the proposed intervention or process improvement is the next step in making an effective business case for quality. It requires using available financial information and making some assumptions to project future expenses related to the project. Financial modeling is covered in more detail in Chapter 10. For the sake of making an effective business case it will suffice to identify all new costs associated with the project over a set period of time, including one-time and recurring operating expenses. For example, the cost of adding additional staff, new equipment, or consultant fees to support the project should be included. The cost of existing internal resources that are reallocated to support the project are typically not factored into the cost estimation of the proposed solution. These types of expenses are considered opportunity costs.

An **opportunity cost** is the financial benefit from using an existing resource for another purpose. For example, a salaried manager spends an average of 20% of her time per week checking accounts receivable. If the business enterprise invests in an automated billing system that cuts in half the amount of time she spends verifying the accounts, assuming her scheduled work time and pay aren't reduced, then the estimated cost from the time she saves is not an actual cost savings. However, if the time saved is re-allocated to other tasks that have a financial impact, such as increasing revenue, then the incremental financial impact should be included in the calculations.

STEP 4. Project the Anticipated Financial Impact

The most challenging step of the process for developing a sound business case is calculating the anticipated financial impact of implementing a proposed performance improvement initiative. The process should include a consistent and conservative method agreed upon by the key stakeholders, including financial leaders. The financial impact should include incremental cost and revenue over a set period, typically 1 to 3 years. Financial impact can be delineated into three types as shown in Exhibit 9.1.

EXHIBIT 9.1

TYPES OF FINANCIAL IMPACT

TYPE	IMPACT	FINANCIAL CHANGE	DEFINITION AND LIMITATION
1	Direct	Decrease expense	Direct measurable impact on a cost center
2	Indirect	Decrease expense	Throughput time saved but no financial impact without reducing expense
3	Indirect	Increase revenue	Throughput time saved but no financial impact without increasing revenue

Type 1: Direct Impact (Decrease Expense)

The first and easiest way to measure the category of financial impact is Type 1. A Type 1 financial impact has a direct effect on reducing operating expense through cutting the acquisition cost of a supply or service, decreasing the amount of the supply or service used, or a combination of both. The financial impact must be measured through the reduction on a financial statement line item for a specific business enterprise. For example, a healthcare provider organization wants to assess the impact of implementing a hip implant demand matching program. Recall from Chapter 7 that demand matching is a provider-driven process to determine the most appropriate implant for the specific needs of each patient. The current cost of waste and the proposed savings using an objective evidence-based clinical algorithm for reducing the number of unnecessary high-demand hips can be calculated as follows:

Type 1 financial impact (demand matching program) = decreased number of high-demand hips (versus low-demand hips) × cost difference between high-demand and low-demand hip implants

= (20% reduction x 400 total high-demand hips per year)

× ($8,500 cost of high-demand implant

− $5,500 cost of low-demand implant)

= (.20 × 400) = 80 high-demand hip reduction

× ($8,500 − $5,500) = $3,000 cost savings per hip implant

= $240,000 annual hip implant savings (current cost of waste)

The total projected financial impact from the demand matching initiative is the same as the current cost of waste assuming there were no incremental costs required to achieve the anticipated savings.

Type 2: Indirect Impact (Decrease Expense)

A Type 2 indirect financial impact results from improving throughput cycle time. The cost savings typically occur from extracting unnecessary labor and non-labor expense from an inefficient process. Similar to Type 1, the financial impact of a Type 2 financial impact is not achieved until it can be allocated to a specific cost center reflected in a financial statement. For example, a business enterprise identifies an opportunity to improve "top of license" use of radiologic technologists by having less expensive patient transporters move patients to and from the emergency department to get a diagnostic study. Collecting some basic historical data combined with conducting a patient flow map and determining the cycle time previously presented produces the information shown in Table 9.6.

The estimated current cost of waste from using more expensive technologists versus patient transporters can be calculated as follows:

| Cost of waste (using radiologic technologists to transport patients) | = number of technologist hours transporting patients × technologist cost per hour
= 1,583 × $27.14
= $42,963 cost savings |

The total potential savings from using less costly patient transporters is the expense of three-quarters of a full-time equivalent (FTE). To complete the calculation, the cost of using patient transporters must be subtracted from the current estimated cost of waste using radiologic technologists. Calculating ROI will be addressed in Step 5.

It's important to note that choosing not to fill an open employee position *is not* an actual cost savings, rather a cost avoidance. A **cost avoidance** does not have a measurable financial impact on the bottom line versus deferring a potential expense. Any incremental cost savings must have a measurable impact on the business enterprise's bottom line. An actual cost reduction can only be recognized when the measurable impact from the initiative affects a cost center. For example, reducing patient LOS only has a financial impact if the "extra" staff time gained, for example, through cutting patient days is reduced from closing a nursing unit or flexing-off employees. The business case for reducing LOS is addressed later. Finally, the success of implementing an initiative with a Type 2 financial impact has two potential gains. Beyond achieving a measurable cost savings from increasing efficiency the business enterprise should also create the potential for additional capacity to grow support volume and market share.

Type 3: Indirect Impact (Increase Revenue)

A Type 3 financial impact occurs when the business enterprise leverages the additional growth capacity achieved from a Type 2 financial impact initiative. Again, the financial impact is only recognized when the additional

TABLE 9.6 Calculating Impact of Reducing Radiologic Technologist Transport Time

Average total time for radiologic technologist to transport patient to and from emergency department (ED; round trip)	9.5 minutes
Total annual ED visits	50,000 patients
Percent of patients requiring a diagnostic study	20%
Number of patients requiring a diagnostic study	10,000 imaging studies
Total time spent transporting patients (annually)	1,583 hours
Hourly rate for radiologic technologist (including benefits)	$27.14
Hourly rate for patient transporter (including benefits)	$11.80

TABLE 9.7 **Calculating Impact of Reducing Patient No-Shows and Cancellations**

Annual outpatient diagnostic imaging volume	32,500 patients
Patient appointment cancellation and no-show rate	20%
Annual number of cancelled and no-show appointments	6,500 appointments
Average net revenue per diagnostic imaging test	$750.00

volume results in incremental revenue noted on a financial statement. Leaders should continuously identify and assess incremental volume and market growth opportunities such as those discussed in Chapter 8, including service recovery. The potential from patients who cancel or no-show at their scheduled appointments creates a double hit to the bottom line resulting from the expense incurred with the decreased labor productivity and also from the lost revenue from the absent patient.

Using the example from the Type 2 financial impact, assume that the three-quarters FTE radiologic technologist cannot be eliminated due to staffing and scheduling intricacies. The business enterprise can translate the additional workload capacity from the saved radiologic technologist time to leverage a potential revenue growth opportunity, by using the 1,583 hours of radiologic technologist time to call patients with a prepared script to remind them of their appointment and answer any questions, such as any special instructions or driving directions. Evidence-based management research has shown that using clinic staff to remind patients of an upcoming appointment can significantly decrease the no-show rate compared to an automated appointment reminder system.[9] Information for projecting the financial impact of the proposed initiative to reduce patient no-shows and cancellations is provided in Table 9.7.

Assuming a targeted 50% reduction of appointment cancellations and no-shows in one year by instituting the patient call reminders using radiologic technologists, the Type 3 financial impact can be calculated as follows:

Type 3 financial impact (decreasing patient no-show and cancellation rate) = targeted annual reduction of cancelled and no-show appointments
× average net revenue per diagnostic imaging test
= (50% × 6,500) × $750

= $2,437,500 annual net revenue increase

STEP 5. Calculate Return on Investment

The final step for making an effective business case is determining the projected gain or ROI from the proposed intervention. **ROI** is simply the financial performance of a project. It is the revenue the business enterprise gets back after paying for all expenses related to the project. Different types of ROI will be covered in Chapter 10. The business case ROI is calculated by dividing the forecasted net financial impact from Step 4 by the cost of the proposed solution from Step 3 as shown in Box 9.6. ROI can also be expressed as a percentage by multiplying the result by 100.

BOX 9.6

CALCULATING RETURN ON INVESTMENT (ROI)

$$ROI = \frac{\text{Anticipated financial impact} - \text{Cost of the proposed solution}}{\text{Cost of proposed solution}}$$

For example, the total cost of a project to improve clinical documentation through dedicated on-site support is $10,000 per month. The additional revenue expected from reducing documentation errors is $12,500 per month. The ROI can be calculated as follow:

$$\text{ROI (improved clinical documentation)} = \frac{\$12,500 - \$10,000}{\$10,000}$$

$$= \frac{\$2,500}{\$10,000}$$

$$= 0.25 \text{ or } 25\% \text{ return on investment}$$

This means that the organization will get back $0.25 (return) for every dollar it plans to spend on the project (investment). The dollar amount ROI can be determined by multiplying the monthly financial impact of $2,500 by 12 months equaling $30,000. The ROI percent does not change. The ROI from a project can be considered the same way as calculating net income or operating margin presented in Chapter 2, where expense is subtracted from revenue.

MONETIZING QUALITY IMPROVEMENT INITIATIVES

Any proposed quality improvement initiative can be translated into a defensible business case. However, as previously presented, the challenge and limitation is projecting the financial impact. Linking quality improvement and financial impact is the key to an effective business case. The select highlighted examples from Table 9.8 will be used to illustrate how to calculate the financial impact of common quality improvement initiatives. Supplemental materials for these examples are available online at Springer Connect (visit connect .springerpub.com/content/book/978-0-8261-4464-5/chapter/ch09 and access the show chapter supplementary dropdown at the beginning of the chapter).

TABLE 9.8 **Monetizing Quality Improvement Initiatives**

QUALITY IMPROVEMENT GOAL	LEADER ACTION(S)	FINANCIAL IMPACT
Reduce healthcare provider organization-acquired infection rate	Adopt infection prevention and control best practice guidelines	Reduce operating expense (labor and non-labor)
Improve documentation and coding accuracy	Implement compliant documentation management program	Increase revenue
Improve care delivery efficiency Reduce average length of stay Reduce left without being seen	Reduce cycle time (outpatient and inpatient)	Reduce operating expense (labor and non-labor) Increase revenue
Reduce patient no-show and cancellation rate	Implement patient call reminders	Reduce operating expense (labor) Increase revenue
Improve inpatient bed utilization	Implement patient acuity-bed match initiative	Reduce operating expense (labor)
Improve patient experience	Implement service recovery initiative	Increase revenue
Reduce provider and staff turnover rate	Increase employee engagement and satisfaction	Reduce operating expense (labor)
Create a new or expand existing program or service	Launch growth plan	Increase revenue

TABLE 9.9 **Financial Impact for Common Hospital-Acquired Conditions**

HOSPITAL-ACQUIRED CONDITION (HAC)	EXCESS COST
CDI (*Clostridium difficile* infection)	$7,766–$11,285
MRSA (methicillin-resistant *Staphylococcus aureus*)	$6,248
SSI (surgical site infection)	$20,785–$23,272
VRE (vancomycin-resistant enteroccoi)	$27,190–$33,251

Source: Fuller RL, McCullough EC, Bao MZ, et al. Estimating the cost of potentially preventable hospital acquired complications. *Health Care Financ Rev*. 2009;30(4):17-32.

Reduce Hospital-Acquired Infection Rate

Healthcare provider organizations are keenly interested in reducing preventable adverse events that impact patient safety, clinical outcomes, and the total cost of care. Patients who acquire an infection during their visit are highly visible through national reporting due to their potential for increased mortality and morbidity. They also reflect significant cost of waste. Table 9.9 shows the range of financial impact for some of the most common acquired conditions that are typically non-reimbursable expenses and without factoring any value-based reimbursement penalties levied by federal and private payers.

With a few pieces of data including the incremental cost per episode, the baseline rate, and the target rate, the potential financial impact from reducing the surgical site infection (SSI) rate, for example, can be calculated as follows:

Baseline SSI rate	2%
Cost per SSI	$20,750
Total annual surgical cases	12,500
Target SSI rate	1%
Cost of waste	= (baseline SSI rate x total annual surgical cases) × cost per SSI
	= (.02 × 12,500) × $20,750
	= $5,187,500 cost of waste
Financial impact (decreasing SSI rate 1%)	= baseline SSI cost of waste − target SSI cost of waste
	= $5,187,500 − [(.01 × 12,500) × $20,750]
	= $5,187,500 − $2,593,750
	= $2,593,750 projected annual cost savings

Improve Documentation and Coding

As presented in Chapter 4 the case mix index (CMI) is an important operations indicator reflecting the diversity, complexity, and resource needs of all the patients in a hospital. A higher CMI means more reimbursement based on documentation and coding completeness and accuracy. There is a tendency to undercode for the services provided out of fear of audits, financial penalties, and being accused of fraud. An example of calculating the potential financial impact from implementing a coding documentation initiative for heart failure, as an example, is as follows:

Medicare base payment rate	$5,797		
	MS-DRG	Relative Weight	Reimbursement
Relative weight and	291w MCC	1.2585	$7,296
reimbursement	292 w CC	1.0134	$5,875
	293 w/o MCC/CC	0.8765	$5,081
Volume and reimbursement	MS-DRG	Volume	Reimbursement
(annual)	291w MCC	50	$364,776
	292 w CC	200	$1,174,936
	293 w/o MCC/CC	150	$762,161
	Total 400 cases		$2,607,811

Cost of waste assuming an audit shows that cases with MCC are
undercoded by 20% and CC are undercoded by 25%

		Change due to CDI initiative	
MS-DRG	Volume	Reimbursement	
291w MCC	10	$22,145	
292 w CC	50	$39,680	
293 w/o MCC/CC	-60		

Financial impact (increasing MCC 10% and CC 25%)	$61,825 projected annual revenue increase

Improve Care Delivery Efficiency (Length of Stay)

Inpatient care comprises nearly one-third of all healthcare expenditures in the United States.[10] Inpatient LOS is an important indicator and good proxy for leaders on how efficiently the healthcare provider organization uses its resources. Optimizing and reducing LOS improves financial, operational, and clinical outcomes. It also can improve patient outcomes by minimizing the risk of hospital-acquired conditions.[11] A shorter LOS is typically better and means relatively lower total cost of care.

The traditional method for determining the financial impact from reducing LOS, for example, can be calculated for total joint replacement as follows:

MD-DRG 470	Total joint replacement
Annual discharges	550
Average length of stay	4.0 days
Annual patient days	2,200 days
Average cost per bed day	$1,500
Geometric LOS (target)	3.0 days
Projected annual patient days	1,650 days

$$\text{Cost of waste} = \text{(current annual patient days x cost per bed day)}$$
$$- \text{(projected annual patient days x cost per bed day)}$$
$$= (2,200 \times \$1,500) - (1,650 \times \$1,500)$$
$$= \$3,300,000 - \$2,475,000$$

Financial impact (reducing LOS 25%) = $825,000 projected annual cost savings (traditional method)

Multiplying the average cost per patient day by the reduced days shown results in the projected $825,000 annual savings using the traditional approach to monetizing LOS. However the projected cost savings is artificially inflated using the traditional approach. As shown in Figure 9.4 the cost of care is typically higher in the beginning of the hospital stay due to the nursing intake and diagnostic testing. The cost of care per day tapers as the patient stay draws near discharge.

Since only the last day of stay is impacted, the LOS reduction should be multiplied by the total cost of the last day of discharge using the cost per patient day shown in Table 9.10.

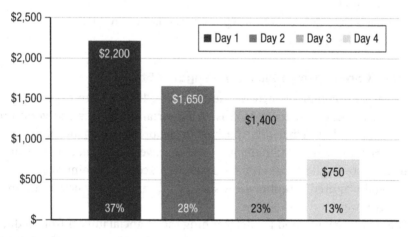

FIGURE 9.4 Cost per patient day.

TABLE 9.10 **Total Cost per Patient Day**

Day	VARIABLE EXPENSE		
	Direct	Indirect	Total
1	$660	$2,200	$1,540
2	$495	$1,650	$1,155
3	$420	$1,400	$980
4	$225	$750	$525
Total	$1,800	$6,000	$4,200

Projected annual last days (Day 4)	550 days
Cost of waste	= projected annual patient days reduction × cost per bed day 4
	= 550 × $525
Financial impact (reducing LOS 20%)	= $288,750 projected annual cost savings (preferred method)

The revised financial impact using only the cost of the last day of care results in significantly reduced savings than estimated using the traditional method, 65% less. Given that the majority of operating expense is from labor, the projected savings can be achieved only by eliminating unnecessary staffing. Otherwise, the capacity created from the Type 2 financial impact can be used to generate additional revenue. The primary opportunity that improving cycle time throughput can address pent up demand is achieving growth goals in the emergency department (ED).

Reduce Emergency Department Left Without Being Seen Rate

ED capacity in the United States has become increasingly stressed as more patients requiring urgent and non-urgent attention seek critical care and the around-the-clock convenience. According to research, a growing population with chronic diseases and fewer hospitals and hospital beds are the primary causes of ED crowding leading to lengthy delays in diagnosis and treatment.[12] An estimated 2.4% of patients who visit an ED eventually leave without being seen or treated.[13] Waiting for an inpatient bed is the common rate-limiting factor in moving patients out of the ED. As an example, the potential financial impact from patients leaving the ED without being seen can be calculated as follows:

Annual ED visits	50,000 visits
ED admission rate	15%
LWOBS current rate	3%
Average net patient revenue:	
Per ED visit (outpatient)	$500
Per ED admission (inpatient)[a]	$2,500
Annual lost ED visits (LWOBS)	1,500 visits
Annual lost ED admissions	225 admissions
Cost of waste	= (current LWOBS rate × annual ED visits) × average net revenue per visit

$$+ [(\text{ED admission rate} \times \text{annual lost ED visits}) \text{ x average net revenue per admission}]$$

$$- (\text{ED visits admitted} \times \text{average net revenue per visit})^b$$

$$= (.03 \times 50{,}000) \times \$500$$

$$+ [(.15 \times 1{,}500) \times \$2{,}500] - (225 \times \$500)$$

$$= \$750{,}000 + \$450{,}000$$

Financial impact
(3% LWOBS) $= \$1{,}200{,}000$ projected annual revenue increase

a. Includes observation admissions.

b. Net revenue per ED visit is included in inpatient reimbursement when the patient is admitted.

The annual total cost of waste in lost revenue from the 3% of patients who left the ED without being seen is $1.2 million. Since it is unrealistic to expect that the left without being seen (LWBS) rate can be reduced to zero, leaders must set a realistic and achievable goal. Reducing the LWBS by 1% over 1 year, for example, results in the following calculations where the cost of waste and potential savings is the difference between the current and target LWBS.

Annual lost ED visits (LWOBS)   1,000 visits

Annual lost ED admissions   150 admissions

Cost of waste $= (\text{target LWOBS rate} \times \text{annual ED visits})$

$\times$ average net revenue per visit

$+ [(\text{ED admission rate} \times \text{annual lost ED visits}) \times \text{average net revenue per admission}]$

$- (\text{ED visits admitted} \times \text{average net revenue per visit})^b$

$= (.02 \times 50{,}000) \times \$500$

$+ [(.15 \times 1{,}000) \times \$2{,}500] - (150 \times \$500)$

$= \$500{,}000 + \$300{,}000 = \$800{,}000$

Financial impact (2% LWOBS) $= \$400{,}000$ projected annual revenue increase

Monitoring Value: Pulling It All Together in the Integrated Dashboard

The leadership imperative to improve value by linking quality and cost is an ongoing process that must be continuously monitored. While quality and cost

EXHIBIT 9.2

INTEGRATED QUALITY AND COST DASHBOARD EXAMPLE

Performance Improvement Initiatives	BASELINE JANUARY 1–DECEMBER 31, 20X1				TARGET BY DECEMBER 31, 20X2			PERFORMANCE JANUARY 1, 20X1–DECEMBER 31, 20X2							
								September		October		November		Year to Date	
	Cases	Rate	Cost per Case	Total Cost of Waste	Cases	Rate	Cost Reduction	Cases	Cost Savings	Cases	Cost Savings	Cases	Cost Savings	Cases	Cost Savings
C. *diff* Infection	84	6.00%	$7,285	$611,940	42	3.0%	$305,970	5	$14,570	9	($14,570)	4	$21,855	68	$116,560
MRSA	43	8.00%	$6,248	$268,664	27	5.0%	$437,360	0	$24,992	1	$18,744	1	$18,744	27	$99,968
SSI	11	4.50%	$23,272	$255,992	5	2.0%	$651,616	1	($23,272)	0	$23,272	1	$0	5	$139,632
LWOBS	900	3.00%	$725	$652,500	750	2.5%	$25,375	83	($5,800)	61	$10,150	53	$15,950	711	$137,025
Re-admissions	78	3.60%	$7,300	$569,400	32	1.5%	$153,300	2	$36,500	2	$36,500	1	$43,800	51	$197,100
Clinic no-shows	341	18.00%	$230	$78,430	208	11.0%	$35,420	26	$460	20	$1,840	13	$3,450	216	$28,750
Total				$2,436,926			$1,609,041		$47,450		$75,936		$103,799		$719,035

are inextricably linked, the performance metrics that leaders use to assess them typically are not. Quality scorecards are often void of the current cost of waste and the potential financial impact from various performance improvement initiatives. Exhibit 9.2 represents how leaders can integrate quality and cost on the same dashboard to enable improved decision-making. Note the ability to assess and prioritize performance improvement initiatives using both quality (leading indicator) and cost (lagging indicator) measures to improve leadership decision-making.

Overcoming Risk Aversion to the Proposed Business Case

The process for developing a sound business case is necessary; however, it does not guarantee approval of the proposed project or initiative. Beyond gaining stakeholder buy-in, a common barrier to leadership approval is a culture of risk aversity caused by financial austerity. Leaders in provider healthcare organizations tend to be very conservative in selecting which projects to pursue and lean toward those with higher and more certain ROIs. What's more, leadership teams often spend too much time developing and weighing all possible options, their implications, and potential implementation challenges rather than testing the impact of an innovative idea. This is commonly referred to as "paralysis by analysis." Notwithstanding the basic human fears of change and failure, leaders are often reluctant to pursue new or untried ideas which leads to avoidance and delays. Forming a committee, deferring to another committee, requesting excessive data, and waiting for a "better time" are all ineffective but not uncommon ways to deflect the need for meaningful change. Using a small, focused pilot is a valuable approach to proof the concept of a novel idea that can accelerate sustainable improvement.

Championed by the Institute for Health Improvement as an extension of the Plan-Do-Study-Act model (Figure 9.5) introduced by Walter Shewart in the 1920s, **rapid cycle testing** is a simple and effective approach to implement a small test of change and observe the impact prior to a potentially time-consuming and costly full implementation.

The steps for conducting a rapid cycle listed in Box 9.7 include identifying what specific measure will be tested, how it will be tested, collecting baseline data, communicating with the key staff and other stakeholders involved, running the test, analyzing the results, and repeating the steps as necessary. As previously shared, at least 30 data points are needed to establish the baseline and assess the test. The results of the test can then be used to prepare a run chart showing the impact of the intervention on the performance measure as shown in Figure 9.6.

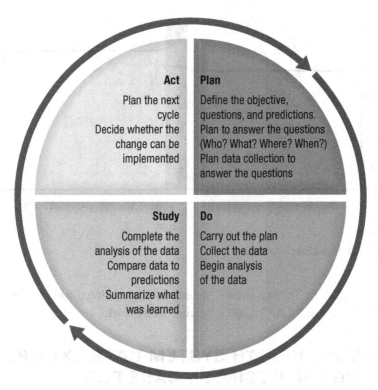

FIGURE 9.5 Plan-do-study-act model for improvement.

BOX 9.7

STEPS FOR CONDUCTING A RAPID CYCLE TEST
1. Identify the measure to test
2. Create a plan to test the change
3. Collect baseline data
4. Engage key stakeholders
5. Run the test
6. Analyze results
7. Repeat the process (as needed)

Based on the degree of success of the rapid cycle test the changes are then permanently hardwired into the process, modified for further testing, or discarded as a bad idea. Discarded ideas should not be considered failures in a negative way; rather, they are an effective way to move along the learning curve

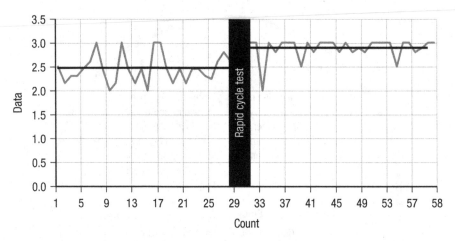

FIGURE 9.6 Run chart example.

toward success. As Thomas Edison stated when inventing the lightbulb: "I have not failed. I've just found 10,000 ways that won't work."

REGIONAL HEALTH SYSTEM CASE EXAMPLE: MAKING THE BUSINESS CASE FOR DECREASING CROSS-CONTAMINATED BLOOD CULTURE SPECIMENS IN THE EMERGENCY DEPARTMENT

Blood culture contamination in the Regional Health System's (RHS) ED has increased steadily over the past year to nearly 5%. Blood culture contamination is a common problem causing unnecessary patient morbidity and increased healthcare costs. EDs are especially susceptible to blood culture contamination with many having contamination rates higher than the 3% benchmark recommended by the Clinical and Laboratory Standards Institute.[14] Lab specimens for blood cultures are typically drawn by the ED nurses. During times when the ED becomes overcrowded and the nurses are busy triaging and treating patients, certified phlebotomists from the lab are used to help draw blood for diagnostic testing. The staff member drawing the lab can be identified by a discrete number to track contaminated specimens.[15]

The Director of the RHS ED was asked by the Chief Medical Officer (CMO) to assess opportunities to address the cross-contamination problem and develop recommendations to improve both the accuracy and cost efficiency of patient diagnostic testing while reducing the cross-contamination rate to the national benchmark of 3% or less within 1 year. However, due to continued

TABLE 9.11 **Number of Contaminated Blood Culture Specimens by Type of Staff Drawing**

MONTH	ED RN STAFF LAB DRAWS		PHLEBOTOMIST LAB DRAWS	
	SPECIMENS DRAWN	NUMBER CONTAMINATED	SPECIMENS DRAWN	NUMBER CONTAMINATED
July	553	23	193	3
August	367	23	139	2
September	386	16	160	4
October	403	22	154	3
November	340	27	158	2
December	383	28	152	5
January	408	26	170	2
February	350	25	138	3
Total	3,190	190	1,264	24
Annualized	4,785	285	1,896	36

financial challenges straining already thin operating margins, the hospital CEO has put a moratorium on any funding for clinical quality improvement initiatives that do not have a positive return. Given the current austere environment and knowing that any meaningful efforts to impact material change will involve unbudgeted resources, the Director begins preparing a business case to present to the hospital executive committee using the data provided in Table 9.11 and the Five Steps for Making an Effective Business Case presented in Box 9.4.

STEP 1. Identify the Performance Improvement Opportunity and Goal

Contamination rates:

Average: 4.89%   RN: 6.06%   Phlebotomist: 1.90%

STEP 2. Calculate the Cost of Waste

Based on the contamination rates for nurses and phlebotomists provided the total annual cost of waste is calculated as follows:

Cost per contamination $5,270

$$= \text{(ED RN staff number of contaminated specimens)} + \text{(phlebotomist number of contaminated specimens)} \times \text{cost per contamination}$$

$$= (285 + 36) \times \$5,270$$

Total cost of waste (annualized) $= \$1,691,670$ projected annual cost from ED cross-contaminated specimens

STEP 3. Determine the Cost of the Proposed Solution

The Director proposed a multi-pronged approach to reducing the cross-contamination rate including providing staff education and training and increasing the use of phlebotomists to allow nurses to focus on more "top of license" tasks. The projected cost for adding phlebotomists to cover a range of staffing options is presented in Table 9.12.

The total number of ED nurses to be trained is 120 using an external consultant at the in-service rate of $55.00 per hour for each nurse. The projected cost for providing education and training ranging from 1 to 4 sessions per year accounts for different shifts, vacations, and staff turnover and is provided in Table 9.13.

STEP 4. Project the Anticipated Financial Impact

Based on the potential range of interventions and their costs the Director develops a sensitivity analysis to identify the total investment required to reduce the cross-contamination rate to 3% or less. More on sensitivity analyses

TABLE 9.12 Phlebotomist Staffing Shifts and Costs

FTE	SHIFTS COVERED	DAYS COVERED	WEEKLY HOURS	ANNUAL HOURS	EXPENSE (INCLUDING BENEFITS)
1.0	1	5	40	2,080	$ 50,180
2.0	2	5	80	4,160	$ 100,360
3.0	3	5	120	6,240	$ 150,540
1.4	1	7	56	2,912	$ 70,252
2.8	2	7	112	5,824	$ 140,504
4.2	3	7	168	8,736	$ 210,756

TABLE 9.13 Nurse Education and Training In-Service Costs

ANNUAL TRAINING SESSIONS	EXPENSE
1	$ 5,400
2	$10,800
3	$16,200
4	$21,600

TABLE 9.14 **Intervention Costs**

PERCENT CHANGE	CONTAMINATED SPECIMENS	CONTAMINATION RATE	COST OF CONTAMINATION	PROJECTED COST REDUCTION
0.0%	327	4.89%	$1,723,290	
−5.0%	311	4.65%	$1,637,126	$86,165
−10.0%	294	4.41%	$1,550,961	$172,329
−15.0%	278	4.16%	$1,464,797	$258,494
−20.0%	262	3.92%	$1,378,632	$344,658
−30.0%	229	3.43%	$1,206,303	$516,987
−40.0%	196	2.94%	$1,033,974	$689,316
−50.0%	164	2.45%	$861,645	$861,645
−60.0%	131	1.96%	$689,316	$1,033,974

will be presented in Chapter 10. The projected financial impact of reducing the cross-contamination rate is presented in Table 9.14.

STEP 5. Calculate the Return on Investment

Assuming the reasonable accuracy of the source data used to project the financial impact of the various combinations and options for reducing the cross-contamination rate summarized in Table 9.14, the Director can make an informed recommendation to the CMO to achieve the goal. There are several key results from the Director's analysis that are worth noting:

1. Current cost of waste is $1,723,290, which is also the cost of doing nothing or the status quo.

2. Breakeven point is between 10% to 15% contaminated specimen reduction. Recall from Chapter 2 the breakeven point is where the total projected cost of the initiative and the expected financial impact are equal. The correlation between reducing cross-contamination and ROI is shown in Table 9.15 and graphically in Figure 9.7.

3. Reducing cross-contamination rate from the current 4.8% average to the goal of 3% or less, the Director must decrease the number of contaminations by 131 in 12 months or 11 per month which would be an ROI of $456,960 (196.7%).

4. Internal best practice benchmark based on the current phlebotomist contamination rate of 1.96% results in $801,618 ROI (345%).

Supplemental materials for the Case Example are available online at Springer Connect (visit connect.springerpub.com/content/book/978-0-8261-4464-5/chapter/ch09 and access the show chapter supplementary dropdown at the beginning of the chapter).

TABLE 9.15 Intervention Costs

	PERCENT CHANGE	CONTAMINATED SPECIMENS	CONTAMINATION RATE	COST OF CONTAMINATION	PROJECTED COST REDUCTION	ROI	PERCENT ROI
①	0.0%	327	4.89%	$1,723,290			
	−5.0%	311	4.65%	$1,637,126	$86,165	−$146,192	−62.9%
②	−10.0%	294	4.41%	$1,550,961	$172,329	−$60,027	−25.8%
	−15.0%	278	4.16%	$1,464,797	$258,494	$26,138	11.2%
	−20.0%	262	3.92%	$1,378,632	$344,658	$112,302	48.3%
	−30.0%	229	3.43%	$1,206,303	$516,987	$284,631	122.5%
	−40.0%	196	2.94%	$1,033,974	$689,316	$456,960	196.7%
③	−50.0%	164	2.45%	$861,645	$861,645	$629,289	270.8%
④	−60.0%	131	1.96%	$689,316	$1,033,974	$801,618	345.0%

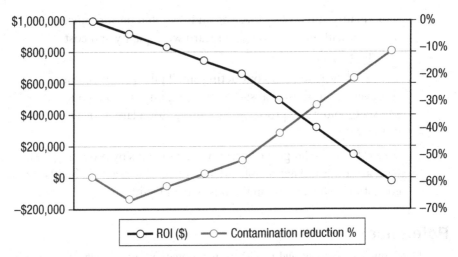

FIGURE 9.7 Contamination reduction return on investment.

SUMMARY

Leaders can use a sound business case as a useful evaluative tool to assess the financial impact of both the current cost of waste and of implementing a proposed intervention. An effective business case is comprehensive yet simple to understand with conservative financial projections to support effective decision-making to take the necessary actions that improve financial and operations performance. There are several methods to reasonably predict the cost of waste and financial impact of a proposed solution including manually, CCR, chart audit, and from published studies. Leaders can use simple process improvement techniques to reduce waste and unnecessary cost including process mapping, cycle time, defining the problem and goal, and rapid cycle testing. Monetizing quality efforts is important to enable assessing and prioritizing performance improvement opportunities.

CALLS TO ACTION

Leaders should:

- Make the business case for quality by adopting a deliberate business case analysis process to assess and prioritize ROI for all performance improvement initiatives.

- Link quality and cost by creating an integrated performance improvement measurement scorecard with quality and cost measures.

- Use rapid cycle tests by conducting small pilots to overcome risk aversion and fiscal austerity and gain buy-in from your key stakeholders by proofing the concept for a larger idea or initiative.

- Break down the language barrier with clinicians by providing them with accurate and actionable financial data and practical hands-on education and training on the business of healthcare.

References

1. Goldsmith J. Hospitals and physicians: not a pretty picture. *Health Aff.* 2006;26(1): w72-w75.
2. Mark TL, Evans W, Schur C, et al. Hospital-physician arrangements and hospital financial performance. *Medical Care.* 1998;36(1):67-78.
3. Shrank WH, Rogstad TL, Parekh N. Waste in the US health care system: estimated costs and potential for savings. *JAMA.* 2019;322(15):1501-1509.
4. Institute of Medicine. *The Healthcare Imperative: Lowering Costs and Improving Outcomes: Workshop Series Summary.* The National Academies Press; 2010.
5. Berwick DM, Hackbarth AD. Eliminating waste in US health care. *JAMA.* 2012;307(14):1513-1516.
6. Brownlee S. The overtreated American. *The Atlantic Monthly.* January/February 2003: 89-91.
7. Daly R. Health care's first cost accounting adoption model is now available. Healthcare Financial Management Association. February 13, 2019. https://www.hfma.org/topics/news/2019/02/63271.html
8. Lawson R. Key findings of the HFMA-IMA initiative. Healthcare Financial Management Association. 2017.
9. Parikh A, Gupta K, Wilson AC, et al. The effectiveness of outpatient appointment reminder systems in reducing the no-show rates. *Am J Med.* 2010;123(6):542-548.
10. Gilbert J. Hospital readmissions and length of stay. [Web blog post]. The Incidental Economist. August 5, 2015. https://theincidentaleconomist.com/wordpress/hospital-readmissions-and-length-of-stay/
11. Moore B, Levit K, Elixhauser A. Costs for hospital stays in the United States, 2012. Agency for Healthcare Research and Quality: Healthcare Cost and Utilization Project. October 2014. https://www.hcup-us.ahrq.gov/reports/statbriefs/sb181-Hospital-Costs-United-States-2012.jsp
12. Moskop JC, Sklar DP, Geiderman JM, et al. Emergency department crowding, part 1—concept, causes, and moral consequences. *Ann Emerg Med.* 2009;53(5):605-611.
13. Li DR, Brennan JJ, Kreshak AA, et al. Patients who leave the emergency department without being seen and their follow-up behavior: a retrospective descriptive analysis. *J Emerg Med.* 2019;57(1):106-113.

14. Self WH, Talbot TR, Paul BR, et al. Cost analysis of strategies to reduce blood culture contamination in the emergency department: sterile collection kits and phlebotomy teams. *Infect Control Hosp Epidemiol.* 2014;35(8):1021-1028.
15. Bekeris LG, Tworek JA, Walsh MK, et al. Trends in blood culture contamination: A College of American Pathologists Q-Tracks study of 356 institutions. *Arch Pathol Lab Med.* 2005;129(10):1222-1225.

CHAPTER 10

EVALUATING THE FINANCIAL IMPACT OF A FUTURE PROJECT

LEARNING OBJECTIVES

- Apply several common techniques for projecting financial impact of potential future projects.
- Assess the impact of a critical variable on the viability of a future project by conducting a sensitivity analysis.
- Explain key risk factors to enact effective mitigating actions.
- Improve organizational performance by transferring internal and external best practices through benchmarking.

TOOLS AND TECHNIQUES

- Discounted cash flow (DCF) analysis
- Financial modeling
- Risk analysis
- Sensitivity analysis
- Benchmarking

KEY TERMS AND CONCEPTS

Time value of money	Timeline
Discounting	Discount rate
Present value (PV)	Weighted average cost of capital (WACC)
Future value (FV)	Cost of capital
Cash outflow	Hurdle rate
Cash inflow	Net present value (NPV)

Internal rate of return (IRR)   Activity-based costing (ABC)

Payback period   Sensitivity analysis

Pro forma   Financial risk

Resource-based costing   Benchmark

INTRODUCTION

Leaders must continuously monitor the current performance and progress of ongoing initiatives. Leaders must also evaluate the projected performance of future potential initiatives to make sure they are in line with strategic goals and financial performance targets. New projects often require allocating scarce resources and involve a degree of financial risk. For example, launching a new clinical service line or building a new ambulatory care center to grow new revenue can have an unfavorable impact on the bottom line if the projected revenue doesn't materialize causing unexpected financial losses. Leaders can plan for a range of financial outcomes using common methods and tools including the discounted cash flow (DCF) analysis, financial modeling, and risk analysis. Leaders can also monitor desired performance and adopt best practices using benchmarking.

TIME VALUE OF MONEY

Effective financial and operations planning requires that the revenue stream associated with a new project or investment be adjusted to compare expected future dollars to current dollars since money also has time value. The **time value of money** is the notion that a dollar in hand today is worth more than a dollar that will be received at some point in the future. This is due to inflation where spending power decreases over time and also that money in hand today can be invested. Ignoring the time value of money can lead to overestimating the forecasted revenue of a project making it appear more financially attractive than it actually is. To apply the time value of money principle consider a choice of being offered $75 today or being given $100 3 years from now assuming an interest rate of 10%. Determining the present value (PV) of a lump sum is known as **discounting** using the formula shown in Box 10.1.

BOX 10.1

CALCULATING PRESENT VALUE

$$\text{Present value} = \frac{\text{Future value}}{(1 + \text{interest rate})^{\text{number of periods}}} \qquad \text{or } PV = \frac{FV_N}{(1 + I)^N}$$

The PV of the $100 to be received in 3 years with a 10% discount rate is calculated as follows:

where FV = $100

$$PV = \frac{100}{(1 + .10)^3}$$

I = 10%

N = 3 years

$$= \frac{100}{(1.331)}$$

$= \$75$ *(rounding to the nearest dollar)*

Therefore the $75 offered today is *the same* as the $100 that would be received in 3 years using a 10% discount rate. Without the benefit of using time value analysis, the $100 in 3 years might be chosen as the preferable option when they are the same.

CONDUCTING A DISCOUNTED CASH FLOW ANALYSIS

Evaluating the expected future value (FV) of cash flow from a potential project requires conducting a **DCF analysis**. The DCF analysis estimates the **present value (PV)** or the value today of the expected **future value (FV)** of the cash flow from an initiative or investment based on making reasonable projections of how much revenue it will generate. The steps for conducting a DCF analysis are listed in Box 10.2.

BOX 10.2

STEPS FOR CONDUCTING A DISCOUNTED CASH FLOW ANALYSIS
STEP 1. Identify cash outflow.
STEP 2. Estimate cash inflow.
STEP 3. Establish discount rate.
STEP 4. Calculate return on investment (ROI).

STEP 1. Determine Cash Outflow

The **cash outflow** is an initial expense required to start or an operating expense to support a project. It can be recurrent operating expenses such as staff salary and supplies or capital expense such as new diagnostic imaging equipment.

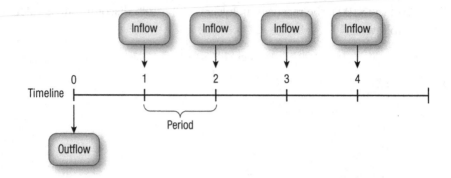

FIGURE 10.1 Cash outflow and cash inflows.

Recall from Chapter 4 that the statement of cash flows reflects cash coming into and leaving the business enterprise.

STEP 2. Estimate Cash Inflow

A **cash inflow** is the anticipated revenue from business operations which can also can be the measurable cost savings from implementing a performance improvement initiative. Estimating patient demand to project expected revenue was addressed in Chapter 9. Financial modeling will be covered later in the chapter. The relationship between cash inflow and cash outflow for a new project is shown on the **timeline** in Figure 10.1, where the project begins at "Year 0" and the distance between each tick mark represents a specified period of time, usually 1 year.

STEP 3. Establish a Discount Rate

The DCF analysis is used to find the PV of expected future cash flows using a specified interest or discount rate. The **discount rate** in the analysis is used to estimate how much the project's future cash flows would be worth in the present. The discount rate can be the **weighted average cost of capital** (WACC), the proportionately weighted cost of capital from different sources such as common stock and bonds. The **cost of capital** is the required minimum return on the investment that is necessary to make a project or investment worthwhile to justify its cost. The cost of capital also establishes a target rate of return that the business enterprise must achieve from a project to satisfy internal financial goals or the lowest acceptable threshold, known as the **hurdle rate**. The cost of capital and the discount rate together help assess whether a prospective project will be profitable.

The discount rate can be used to compare the financial feasibility and attractiveness across multiple competing projects since resources can only be applied to one project at a time at the expense of pursuing other projects. The discount rate typically reflects the degree of confidence leaders have in a project's future cash flow. The higher the discount rate the more cash flow a project has to generate in order for it to be financially feasible. The greater the risk and uncertainty in the financial projections usually means a higher discount rate. Alternatively, a lower expected risk of the project achieving its financial targets typically warrants a lower discount rate. In normal economic times discount rates are usually between 8% and 14%.

STEP 4. Calculate Return on Investment

There are three basic ways to evaluate the financial viability or return on investment (ROI) of a future project: net present value (NPV), internal rate of return (IRR), and payback approach. All three techniques should be used together to generate a comprehensive picture of a project's potential financial viability or profitability.

Net Present Value

The **NPV** helps to assess the financial feasibility of a project. NPV is the sum of all the PVs of the future cash flows for a project. It is the net cash flow or revenue minus all operating expense for each future time period of the planned project. Calculating NPV requires taking the sum of the calculated expected FVs and applying the established discount rate established in Step 3.

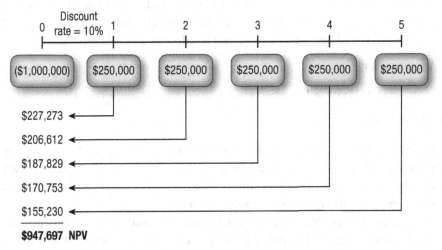

FIGURE 10.2 Calculating net present value (NPV) using a 10% discount rate.

To illustrate how to calculate NPV assume a healthcare provider organization is considering purchasing a new CT scanner that costs $1 million. The new scanner is expected to generate future cash flows minus the operating expenses, such as staffing and supplies of $250,000 per year for the first 5 years. The project is considered to be relatively high risk due to the saturated market for diagnostic imaging so the discount rate is set at 10%. The NPV of the projected future cash flows can be illustrated using the timeline shown in Figure 10.2. The forecasted net revenue for each future year of the project is discounted to the present using the 10% interest rate.

The PVs of the projected future cash flows from the project can be calculated using the previous formula as follows:

$$PV = \frac{FV}{(1+i)^N}$$

$$NPV = \frac{\$250,000}{(1+.10)^1} + \frac{\$250,000}{(1+.10)^2} + \frac{\$250,000}{(1+.10)^3} + \frac{\$250,000}{(1+.10)^4} + \frac{\$250,000}{(1+.10)^5}$$

$$= \$227,273 + \$206,612 + \$187,829 + \$170,753 + \$155,230$$

NPV = $947,697

The NPV of $947,697 is the sum of all future expected cash flows net of operating expenses discounted to the PV using the rate of 10%. Without applying the time value of money using the NPV calculations the projected revenue from the project would be overestimated by approximately $52,000 or more than 5%. NPV can also be calculated using the instructions for Excel worksheets provided in Appendix J. Calculating the NPV factors the net revenue minus expenses for each year and must also account for the initial investment or cash outflow. Therefore the $1 million initial investment must be subtracted from the NPV to determine the ROI and is calculated as follows:

NPV = $947,697

    − ($1,000,000) *cash outflow to purchase the CT scanner in Year 0*

ROI = ($52,303)

The ROI for the project is negative, meaning that it is expected to lose money by the end of the fifth year. Leaders must then determine if the project will be pursued based on the organization's mission and strategic goals relative to other competing interests given scarce resources.

Using the example of purchasing the CT scanner, assume the leadership now has a higher degree of confidence in the project with assumed relatively lower

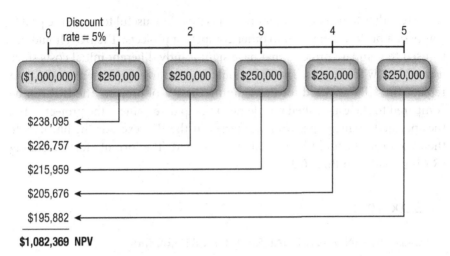

FIGURE 10.3 Calculating net present value (NPV) using a 5% discount rate.

financial risk due to high market demand and low competition. The same process of discounting the future cash flows to the present is done as illustrated in Figure 10.3 and provided using the Excel formula in Appendix J.

The lower expected project risk allows the discount rate to be set at 5% requiring less future cash flow to achieve a higher NPV and ROI, calculated as follows:

$$NPV = \frac{\$250,000}{(1+.05)^1} + \frac{\$250,000}{(1+.05)^2} + \frac{\$250,000}{(1+.05)^3} + \frac{\$250,000}{(1+.05)^4} + \frac{\$250,000}{(1+.05)^5}$$

$$= \$238,095 + \$226,757 + \$215,959 + \$205,676 + \$195,882$$

$$NPV = \$1,082,369$$

$$ROI = \$1,082,369 - (\$1,000,000)$$

$$= \$82,369$$

Without applying the time value of money using the NPV calculations the projected revenue from the project would be misrepresented and underestimated by approximately $82,000 or nearly 7%.

Internal Rate of Return

Another way to evaluate the ROI for a potential project is the IRR. The **IRR** is sometimes referred to as the economic rate of return and is the rate of growth a project is expected to generate. It is the discount rate at which the PV of the costs of a project is equal to the PV of its expected revenue or the rate that produces a NPV of zero. A higher IRR means a higher NPV. The IRR is expressed as a rate rather than a dollar amount and is therefore useful to relate the profitability of a project compared to other competing projects. The IRR should not be used to compare projects that have significantly different initial costs since it would skew the results. The IRR should be used to complement rather than replace the NPV method for determining the PV of project. The IRR can be compared to the established hurdle rate to help determine if the project meets the specified financial performance target. If the IRR exceeds the hurdle rate then the project should be favorably considered. The formula for calculating IRR is provided in Box 10.3.

BOX 10.3

CALCULATING INTERNAL RATE OF RETURN (IRR)

$$NPV = 0 = \text{Cash flow (CF)}_0 + \frac{CF_1}{(1 + IRR)} + \frac{CF_2}{(1 + IRR)^2} + \frac{CF_3}{(1 + IRR)^3} \ldots$$

Consider the same example used in the previous application for determining NPV where the discount rate is set at 5% to calculate the IRR. Calculating the IRR can be done using a financial calculator or using the instructions for the Excel worksheet provided in Appendix J. The IRR for the CT scanner is 7.9%. The IRR for the CT scanner project using either a 5% or 10% discount rate is the same.

Payback Approach

A final way to assess the ROI is the payback approach. The **payback period** is the length of time it takes to get back the initial cost of a new project using expected future cash flows. While the payback approach is easy to understand and use, it does not consider the time value of money. Using the CT scanner example to determine the payback period, Figure 10.4 shows the timeline with

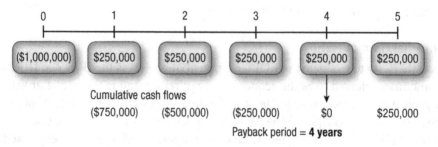

FIGURE 10.4 Calculating payback period.

TABLE 10.1 **Calculating Payback Period**

YEAR	EXPECTED NET CASH FLOWS	PROGRESS TOWARD PAYBACK	
0	($1,000,000)	($1,000,000)	
1	$250,000	($750,000)	
2	$250,000	($500,000)	
3	$250,000	($250,000)	
4	$250,000	$0	Payback at 4 years
5	$250,000	$250,000	

cash outflow, inflows, and the cumulative cash flows over the 5 year life of the project.

The payback period when the organization will recoup the cost of its investment in the CT scanner is 4 years when the cumulative sum of the cash outflow and inflows is zero. Another way to present the payback period approach is shown in Table 10.1.

Limitations of Discounted Cash Flow Analysis

The DCF analysis is critical to estimate the current value of future projected revenue from a project, however it has several limitations. The main limitation is that it requires making assumptions that can impact estimated future cash flows. Estimating future cash flows relies on a number of potentially unforeseeable factors such as shifts in market demand and the status of the economy. Overestimating future cash flows could result in selecting a project that might not pay off and affect the financial performance of the business enterprise. Underestimating cash flows could make the project appear costly and result in a missed opportunity. Selecting the right discount rate also involves a degree of risk and uncertainty that could impact the analysis. Risk analysis and mitigation are addressed later in the chapter.

FINANCIAL MODELING

Developing a reasonable financial forecast of a future project is essential to effective leadership decision-making. Estimating the financial impact of a project involves making key assumptions about expected volume, revenue, and expense. A common challenge for healthcare leaders is failing to use realistic assumptions to forecast revenue and expense, which can impact developing an accurate financial picture of a potential initiative. **Financial modeling** is the deliberate process for creating as accurate a forecast as possible of a project's expected revenue and expense.

DEVELOPING THE FINANCIAL PRO FORMA

The most commonly used aspect of financial modeling is the pro forma. A **pro forma** is a financial statement with projected financial performance based on expectations about the anticipated volume activity, revenue, and expenses. Developing the pro forma is critical to assessing and ultimately monitoring the financial performance of a project. It should therefore involve multidisciplinary stakeholders including clinical, operations, financial, and business intelligence. The timeline of a pro forma is typically 3 to 5 years beginning with "Year 0" when the project starts. The expectations of the predicted financial performance become less certain the further out the pro forma is developed. Exhibit 10.1 presents a simple pro forma showing operating statistics from which revenue and expense assumptions are calculated to determine the expected profitability or net income. Note that the one-time start-up or capital expense is listed separately below operating expense.

Techniques for Allocating Expense

There are two basic approaches leaders can use to allocate costs for projecting the financial impact of a new project: resource-based and activity-based costing. **Resource-based costing** is a holistic way to estimate all of the costs of a proposed project. All costs included in the project are categorized into three areas: implementation, operating, and change as shown in Table 10.2. Expected costs from acquisition and implementation known as start-up costs are typically one-time expenses while the costs from ongoing and continuous operations are usually recurrent costs. The costs associated with anticipated changes such as planned growth or expansion can be both one-time and recurring. Grouping costs into these separate categories is an effective way to identify, analyze, and communicate the cost components of the financial model.

The second method to allocate project expense is **activity-based costing (ABC)**. ABC has been used in manufacturing for decades and attempts to assign costs to discrete activities so that total costs can be better understood and managed. Discrete activities could include the cost of a specific diagnosis, clinic visit, or surgical procedure. A time-driven ABC though not widespread has significant potential to reduce waste and unnecessary expense and improve accountability with more accurate financial data.[1] ABC is also consistent with many performance improvement techniques aimed at standardizing processes, improving them, and eliminating unnecessary variance. ABC has the potential to better integrate clinical and financial outcomes.

EXHIBIT 10.1

SAMPLE PRO FORMA

	12/31/20X1	12/31/20X2	12/31/20X3
Outpatient clinic visits	40	225	350
Admissions	5	34	53
Charge per outpatient clinic visit	$225	$236	$248
Charge per admission	$10,500	$11,025	$11,576
Gross Revenue	$59,400	$425,250	$694,575
Net Patient Revenue			
Net patient revenue per clinic visit	$113	$118	$124
Net patient revenue per admission	$3,465	$3,638	$3,820
Total Net Patient Revenue	$21,132	$149,369	$243,969
Operating Expenses			
Salary, wages, and benefits	$0	$100,300	$104,312
Supplies	$0	$3,625	$3,806
Marketing	$3,500	$1,500	$1,500
Total Operating Expense	$3,500	$105,425	$109,618
Start-up costs	($18,500)		
Net Income	($868)	$43,944	$134,351

SENSITIVITY ANALYSIS

An important part of financial modeling is understanding the impact of key variables on the projected financial performance of a project. A **sensitivity analysis** is a practical technique leaders can use to identify and assess "what if" scenarios to determine the impact of changes in a key input variable on the

TABLE 10.2 Resource-Based Cost Model

IMPLEMENTATION EXPENSES	OPERATING EXPENSES	CHANGE EXPENSES
Initial start-up costs	Day-to-day operating costs	Planned change costs (growth, reconfiguration)
One-time expenses	Ongoing and recurrent	One-time and recurrent
Site planning, installation, equipment, licensure	Staffing, supplies, leases, depreciation (capital)	Renovation, additional staffing, facilities

bottom line, such as patient volume. Conducting a sensitivity analysis involves changing an input value of the model to observe the effect on the output value. For example, while it's easy to comprehend that decreasing clinic patient volume will likely reduce net revenue, it's important for leaders to be able to project what level of volume is attributed to what amount of revenue to support effective planning and management.

Understanding the range of potential financial outcomes based on input variables is useful to avoid or mitigate the effects of unanticipated changes that can occur either within the organization or in the broader external environment. To illustrate how to apply the sensitivity analysis, consider assessing the financial impact of increasing capacity at an outpatient clinic by expanding physical space and adding providers and staff. As with many business enterprises, the capital for expanding must come from operations. The expense and revenue assumptions for the sensitivity analysis are as follows:

Net revenue per clinic visit: $113

Variable expense per clinic visit
Direct (labor and non-labor) $53
Indirect (marketing) $5

Total operating expense: $58

Net income per clinic visit: $55

Fixed expense (per month): $1,389   *Year 1: $50,000 initial investment for new equipment depreciated over 3 years*

The sensitivity analysis showing the changes in the overall financial impact or net income based on varying volume of clinic visits is presented in Table 10.3.

TABLE 10.3 **Sensitivity Analysis for Clinic Visits**

ADDITIONAL CLINIC VISITS PER MONTH	ADDITIONAL NET REVENUE		TOTAL FINANCIAL IMPACT (ANNUAL)
	MONTHLY	ANNUALLY	
50	$2,750	$33,000	($17,000)
75	$4,125	$49,500	($500)
100	$5,500	$66,000	$16,000
125	$6,875	$82,500	$32,500
150	$8,250	$99,000	$49,000

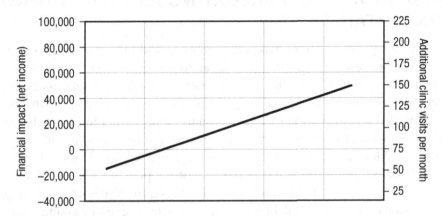

FIGURE 10.5 Sensitivity analysis graph for clinic visits.

The sensitivity analysis can be graphed as shown in Figure 10.5 to assess the projected profitability of the clinic at different levels of volume considering the $50,000 required initial cost. The breakeven point to justify the additional expense occurs at approximately 75 additional clinic visits per month with increasing profitability as the number of visits increase.

NON-FINANCIAL CONSIDERATIONS

The last topic for developing the pro forma involves non-quantitative considerations that are important to evaluating a project. Making a compelling financial case to proceed with a particular project is essential. However, there are other non-financial factors that leaders should consider and factor into their decision-making process. The value of a project based on the healthcare provider organization's mission and strategic goals must be weighed against the projected financial return, either positive or negative. A sound financial return should be used as only one data point when evaluating the viability of a potential new project. Leaders must try to balance the competing needs for fewer resources in their organizations through creating and strengthening strong relationships with key stakeholders, both internal and external. While there may not be a compelling financial case to pursue a particular project, it can still be viable based on supporting other needs, such as increasing the health of underserved populations, regulatory or compliance needs, or supporting long-term strategic growth.

RISK ANALYSIS: EVALUATING AND MITIGATING UNCERTAINTY

Any future project requires making assumptions and therefore involves some degree of uncertainty and risk. **Financial risk** is present whenever there is some chance of earning a return on an investment that is less than projected or required. In general the greater the probability of a result being less than what is projected the greater the risk. Leaders must understand the risk relative to the required return. However, financial analysis alone is not sufficient to predict or achieve anticipated outcomes such as projected cash inflows. Leaders should objectively identify and evaluate all of the potential risks for doing a particular project, the risks of not doing the project, and also how to disengage if the project is unsuccessful. Leaders can begin assessing risk by asking several critical questions listed in Box 10.4.

BOX 10.4

BASIC RISK ANALYSIS QUESTIONS

1. What are the risks of doing the project?
2. What are the risks if the project is accepted and it isn't successful?
3. What is the exit strategy and costs if the project must be abandoned?
4. What are the risks of *not doing* the project?

Leaders should formally assess the risk involved with a potential project *before* it is approved. **Risk analysis** allows preparing contingency plans to mitigate the impact of unintended consequences identified during the analysis. The four primary considerations for conducting a risk analysis and examples of each are presented in Table 10.4. They include determining the critical success factors to achieve the financial or operating targets, identifying the risk factors that need to be continuously monitored, estimating the likelihood of the risk

TABLE 10.4 **Project Risk Factor Analysis**

CRITICAL SUCCESS FACTORS	RISK FACTORS	LIKELIHOOD OF OCCURRING	MITIGATING ACTIONS
• Volume decrease • Reimbursement cut • Operating expense increase	• Demographic shift (decrease in patient target market population) • Entry of new competitor to market	• Low: 1%-30%, • Medium: 31%-60% • High: 61%-100%	• Market share growth (marketing, referral development) • Improve service and access • Decrease expense • Exit the market

occurring, and developing contingency plans if they do occur to avoid or lessen the impact of each risk.

For example, the success of a new clinic under consideration is dependent upon achieving the volume targets specified in the project pro forma. The critical success factor is the clinic volume which could be impacted by an aggressive competitor moving into the market and taking away anticipated volume. Based on market intelligence the likelihood of the competitor entering the market is high, between 70% and 80%. Therefore leaders considering the project would identify and plan for mitigating solutions such as launching a marketing campaign differentiating clinic access and service compared to the competitor.

BENCHMARKING FINANCIAL AND OPERATIONS PERFORMANCE

Leaders should continuously monitor the impact of their performance improvement initiatives compared to their own internal best practices and also those of recognized top-performing organizations through benchmarking. **Benchmarking** is a common process where the healthcare provider organization compares select outcome measures to the "best in class" with the goal of understanding what practices can be adapted or adopted to improve performance. A **benchmark** is simply a standard or target against which performance can be compared or assessed. Benchmarking enables an evidence-based management approach for striving to be *the* best versus better than last year or the best in a limited field.

A common limitation to effective benchmarking is transferring an identified best practice from the benchmarked organization rather than just comparing performance measures. In other words, collecting and reporting benchmark data is often viewed as a means to an end rather than a continuous improvement process where organizations can often disregard the "how" to improving performance. Unlike many industries that closely guard their proprietary best practices most leaders in the healthcare industry support sharing information and best practices that improve health outcomes for the common good. For example, national quality organizations such as the Institute for Health Improvement (IHI) and National Committee for Quality Assurance (NCQA) facilitate sharing ways to transfer best practices. See Box 10.5 for the five steps of benchmarking.

BOX 10.5

FIVE STEPS FOR BENCHMARKING
STEP 1. Determine what to benchmark.
STEP 2. Identify current performance measurement.
STEP 3. Select the right partner.
STEP 4. Examine best practice processes.
STEP 5. Adopt or adapt best practices.

The benchmarking process begins with determining the performance measure to be improved. Next, establishing an accurate performance measurement baseline is necessary to support identifying the gap and goal. The next critical step is selecting the right partner against which to benchmark. The ideal partner can either be from an internal or external best practice. Internal best practices should not be overlooked since they provide credible comparisons with the same common factors affecting performance such as leadership, staffing, processes, and facilities. For example, given two or more providers in the same organizational setting who are performing the same procedure allows useful comparisons such as clinical outcomes, cost, and patient experience. Provider peer-to-peer profiling of internal best practices can be a powerful catalyst for change and performance improvement.

External best practices can be from a nationally-ranked organization that is open to sharing information, which is the next step. Best practices from top-performing organizations can usually be found through publicly available sources such as white papers, peer-reviewed journals, and national conference presentations. A personal or professional network contact can be a good resource to reveal how the organization achieved its desired performance level. Consultants can also be a useful source for identifying and mapping best practices. Lastly, the most important step involves leaders engaging the key stakeholders to develop and implement the plan to map the best practice processes to their organization.

TABLE 10.5 **Healthcare Benchmark Sources**

BENCHMARK TYPE	SOURCE
National safety and quality outcomes	Agency for Healthcare Research and Quality (AHRQ) Leapfrog Hospital Quality and Safety Survey Centers for Medicare & Medicaid Services (CMS) Hospital Compare (Health and Human Services) Becker's Hospital Review
Patient experience	Hospital Compare (Health and Human Services) Press Ganey Associates Health Care Satisfaction Report
Financial performance	Healthcare Financial Management Association (HFMA) American Hospital Directory Becker's Hospital Review American Hospital Association Moody's Investors Service S&P Global Ratings Kaiser State Health Facts
Physician practice operations	Medical Group Management Association (MGMA)
Compensation	Integrated Healthcare Strategies National Healthcare Leadership Compensation Survey
Public health outcomes and rankings	Centers for Disease Control and Prevention (CDC)

To illustrate how to apply benchmarking to improve the patient experience, the Mayo Clinic in Rochester, Minnesota, is consistently ranked among the top-performing healthcare provider organizations in the world. A recent article published in the Mayo Clinic Proceedings[2] contains instructive insight on improving patient experience scores by focusing on how care teams interact with patients about medications, their conditions, and follow-up care needs. Researching best practices to understand the "how" behind the "what" is critical to effective benchmarking. There are numerous publicly available sources[3] for finding the right benchmark and potential partners to improve organizational performance with a representative list provided in Table 10.5.

REGIONAL HEALTH SYSTEM CASE EXAMPLE: PROJECTED FINANCIAL IMPACT OF THE WEEKEND OPERATING ROOM

The Director of Surgical Services is always seeking new opportunities for increasing access to care while adding additional revenue. The Director was approached by an orthopedic surgeon in the community to consider doing elective outpatient surgical cases on the weekend due to a backlog at a competing surgical center in the community where the surgeon currently works. The surgeon has a great reputation for doing high-quality work with excellent outcomes. She is also well-regarded among both her peers and her patients. Offering the surgeon operating room time on the weekend could potentially lead to her increasing caseload during the week since there is capacity. Since Regional Health System (RHS) doesn't currently do weekend elective cases and the surgeon would require additional equipment, staffing, and supplies not presently available, the Director presents the opportunity to the CFO.

The RHS CFO is willing to consider running a weekend elective operating room as long as it doesn't lose money since the operating margins across the system have been declining steadily over the past 2 years. Due to financial constraints the CFO wants to make sure that the additional weekend cases would cover direct and indirect variable costs plus generate enough incremental revenue to pay for the required capital equipment within 3 years *and* meet the organization's 8% hurdle rate for new projects within 3 years. The CFO asks the Director to evaluate the 3-year financial impact of adding the new weekend surgical cases, factoring the cost of the new equipment, by conducting the following analyses and making a recommendation to the executive leadership team:

- DCF analysis
- NPV with projected cash outflow and inflows
- ROI
- Payback period of the capital equipment
- Sensitivity analysis of incremental surgical case volume
- Non-financial considerations
- Risk analysis

The Director gathers the following data and information to make her assumptions for the financial model:

VOLUME AND REVENUE (CASH INFLOW) ASSUMPTIONS

Expected annual case volume:	Low	Medium	High	
	72	84	96	
	Surgeon expects to do 6-8 outpatient surgery cases per month and agrees to postpone cases unless at least two are scheduled.			
	Assume 10% growth in Years 2 and 3			

Charge per case:	$7,500	Based on operating room, anesthesia, and post-anesthesia care unit fee schedule for a basic procedure
Net patient revenue per case:	$3,750	Contractual discount is 50% based on surgeon's payer mix

Expense (Cash Outflow) Assumptions

One operating room is required for the cases. The average case time is 1 hour from cut-to-close. The labor expense rate per hour includes fringe benefits. Weekend staff are guaranteed a minimum of 4 hours regardless of the number of cases. Staffing expense detail is provided in Table 10.6.

TABLE 10.6 **Staffing Expense**

STAFFING REQUIRED	FTE	HOURS	RATE PER HOUR	OVERTIME DIFFERENTIAL	TOTAL RATE	TOTAL STAFFING EXPENSE
Operating room nurse	1.50	8.0	$38.30	$19.15	$57.45	$459.60
Operating room scrub tech	1.00	8.0	$26.30	$13.15	$39.45	$315.60
Recovery room nurse	1.00	8.0	$37.30	$18.65	$55.95	$447.60
Same day surgery nurse	1.25	10.0	$36.30	$18.15	$54.45	$544.50
Total	4.75	34.0				$1,767.30

FTE, full-time equivalent.

Staffing expense per case:	$1,767	
Supply expense per case:	$875	Disposable medical supplies
Purchased services:	$450	Anesthesia cost per case
Capital equipment (start-up) cost:	$75,286	New laparoscopic equipment and instruments to be depreciated over 3 years

Using the low end of the potential volume range for the first year and increasing it by 10% each year the weekend operating room initiative loses

EXHIBIT 10.2

WEEKEND OPERATING ROOM PRO FORMA

	12/31/20X1	12/31/20X2	1231/20X3
Outpatient surgery cases	72	79	87
Charge per outpatient surgery case	$7,500	$7,875	$8,269
Gross Revenue	$540,000	$623,700	$720,374
Net patient revenue			
Net patient revenue per case	$3,750	$3,938	$4,134
Total Net Patient Revenue	$270,000	$311,850	$360,187
Operating expenses			
Salary, wages, and benefits	$127,224	$131,868	$145,055
Supplies	$72,000	$79,200	$87,120
Purchased services	$24,840	$27,324	$30,056
Total Operating Expense	$224,064	$238,392	$262,231
Start-up costs	($75,286)		
Net Income	**($29,350)**	**$73,458**	**$97,956**

approximately $29,000 the first year due to the required capital equipment investment and is profitable in years 2 and 3 as shown in the pro forma in Exhibit 10.2. Subtracting total operating expense from total net patient revenue is required to calculate the NPV of the expected future cash flows presented in Figure 10.6.

The NPV analysis using the discount rate, which is the RHS cost of capital or hurdle rate of 8%, results in the PV of the expected 3-year cash flows of $182,272.

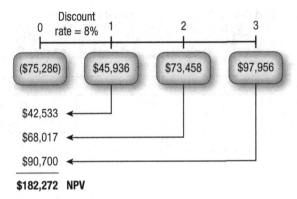

FIGURE 10.6 Weekend operating room net present value (NPV).

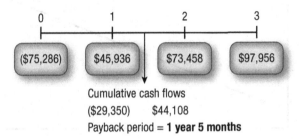

FIGURE 10.7 Weekend operating room payback period.

Return on Investment

Subtracting the start-up cost of the proposed project from the NPV results in the following calculations to determine the ROI:

NPV = $182,272

ROI = $182,272 − ($75,286)

= $106,986

The 3-year ROI is $106,986.

Payback Period

Considering the projected cash flows from offering the weekend operating room the initial capital expense will be recouped within 17 months as shown in Figure 10.7.

TABLE 10.7 **Weekend Operating Room Sensitivity Analysis**

ADDITIONAL CASES PER YEAR	ADDITIONAL NET REVENUE	TOTAL FINANCIAL IMPACT (ANNUAL)
25	$15,950	($59,336)
50	$31,900	($43,386)
75	$47,850	($27,436)
125	$79,750	$4,464
150	$95,700	$20,414

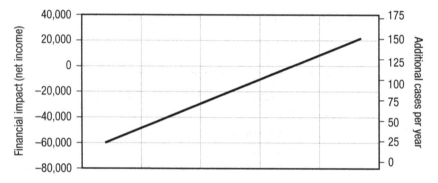

FIGURE 10.8 Weekend operating room sensitivity analysis graph.

SENSITIVITY ANALYSIS

The sensitivity analysis can be graphed as shown in Figure 10.8 to assess the projected profitability of the additional weekend operating room cases at different levels of volume considering the $75,286 initial capital investment. The breakeven point to justify the additional expense occurs at approximately 125 additional cases in year 1 (see also Table 10.7).

NON-FINANCIAL CONSIDERATIONS

Among the non-quantitative considerations that should be factored into the Director's evaluation and recommendation to pursue the weekend operating room project is the potential negative perception among current RHS providers of allocating scarce resources to a surgeon who does not presently have a relationship with the organization, especially if the anticipated volume and revenue don't materialize. Also, leaders should consider how offering the new procedures could impact the organization's safety and quality goals, given the

TABLE 10.8 **Project Risk Factor Analysis**

CRITICAL SUCCESS FACTORS	RISK FACTORS	LIKELIHOOD OF RISK OCCURRING	MITIGATING ACTIONS
• Case volume	• Surgeon is unable or unwilling to deliver volume • Patient payer mix	• Medium: 40%	• Periodic meetings to keep surgeon engaged • Use equipment purchase to grow other volume • Equipment salvage value

potential learning curve for staff. Lastly, leaders should engage key stakeholders such as the governing board, medical staff leaders, and operational staff who will be most impacted by the decision.

Risk Analysis

The primary risk of pursuing the weekend operating room project is the potential for not achieving the targeted volume which is dependent upon a new surgeon. If no additional volume materializes the organization could lose the cost of the capital equipment. The risks of not pursuing the project are the potential lost incremental revenue and the opportunity for RHS to develop a relationship with a new provider. Potential actions that could be taken to mitigate the risks of pursuing the project are listed in Table 10.8 and include making sure the access and service standards for the surgeon's patients meet or exceed her expectations to sustain or increase her engagement and volume.

Given the comprehensive financial and risk analyses, the Director proposes that RHS pursue the weekend operating room project.

The Excel template available on Springer Connect (visit connect.springerpub .com/content/book/978-0-8261-4464-5/chapter/ch10 and access the show chapter supplementary dropdown at the beginning of the chapter) provides a new project evaluation pro forma with the sensitivity analysis that can be modified and used to evaluate other potential new projects.

SUMMARY

Leaders can use the DCF analysis applying the time value of money to forecast the PV of cash flow from a potential future project. Determining reasonably accurate financial projections to support effective leadership decision-making requires modeling through making revenue and cost assumptions using a pro forma. Leaders must evaluate potential risks in assessing the financial viability of future projects and prepare plans to mitigate the impact of unintended consequences. Benchmarking is another effective method leaders can use to monitor project performance compared to internal and external best practices.

CALLS TO ACTION

Leaders should:

- Evaluate the financial impact of potential future projects using common techniques including the DCF analysis, NPV, IRR, and payback method.

- Assess the impact of a key variable such as volume on profitability using a sensitivity analysis.

- Conduct a formal risk analysis before a project is approved to understand and plan for potential factors that could limit or prevent achieving the goals.

- Improve performance using benchmarking to identify and transfer internal and external best practices.

References

1. Kaplan RS, Witkowski ML, Abbott M, et al. Using time-driven activity-based costing to identify value-improvement opportunities in healthcare. *J Healthc Manag.* 2014;59(6): 399-413.
2. Philpot LM, Khokhar BA, DeZutter MA, et al. Creation of a patient-centered journey map to improve the patient experience: a mixed methods approach. *Mayo Clin Proc.* 2019;3(4):466-475.
3. Shoemaker W. Benchmarking boon: tapping publicly available data to improve performance. *Healthcare Financial Management.* 2011;65(6):88-94.

Glossary

Activity-based costing (ABC) assigns costs to discrete activities

Adjusted length of stay reflects patient mix and acuity (how sick patients are)

Asset management ratios measures if a business enterprise has the right amount of resources and how efficiently it is using them

Average daily census (ADC) measures inpatient volume based on the number of patients or occupied beds, typically counted at midnight; also **census**

Balance sheet financial statement showing the business enterprise's assets, liabilities, and owner's equity showing financial performance at a particular point in time, typically at the end of an accounting period or fiscal year

Basic accounting equation assets equals liabilities plus net assets (owner's equity)

Benchmark standard or target against which performance can be compared or assessed to "best in class"

*Benchmarking process where the business enterprise compares specific performance measures to the "best in class" with the goal of understanding what practices can be adapted or adopted

Best and final offer (BAFO) last proposal submitted by vendors competing to provide a product or service

Breakeven point where total revenue minus total expense equals zero; also **breakeven point**

*Breakeven analysis estimates the amount of volume required to recover all expenses associated with a business enterprise, service, program, or project with zero profit

Budget planning document used to establish guidance for managing and monitoring financial performance; also **plan**

Bundled payment fixed payment for an episode of care such as a total joint replacement

Business case evaluative tool to forecast the financial impact and feasibility of a project and support informed leadership decision-making

*Business case analysis evaluative tool to assess the financial impact and feasibility of a project

Capacity total amount of patient volume that can be handled given the desired access and service standards

*Capacity analysis process to assess ability to handle patient volume according to specified service standards

Capital budget allocation of resource expenditures for high-dollar threshold items, such as new equipment and facilities typically, for more long-term strategic goals

---

* Use of this Tool or Technique is described in the book.

Capitation reimbursement model based on a negotiated payment amount per covered life, such as a member of an accountable care organization

Case mix index (CMI) measures the average relative weight and summation of all of the hospital's **Medicare severity-diagnosis related group** (MS-DRG) inpatient discharges

Cash budget projected annual cash based on anticipated revenue cycle performance

Cash inflow anticipated revenue from business operations which can also can be the measurable cost savings from implementing a performance improvement initiative

Cash outflow initial expense or investment required to start a project or operating expense to support it

Charge amount of money billed to a payer for services; also **gross charge, gross revenue, price,** or **fee**

Charge data master (CDM) single standard schedule of fees charged to payers for services

Comparative analysis used to assess performance compared to peer organizations within the same system or against competitors

Competitive differentiation features that set the business enterprise apart from others in the market, such as service, access, and the perception of quality

Competitor entity that offers the same or similar service within the same market as the business enterprise

***Competitor analysis** process to identify and systematically assess market competitors to delineate how the business enterprise can better meet customers' needs

Contractual adjustment difference between the billed charge and the negotiated contractual rate for services; also **discount** or **write off**

Contribution margin financial performance indicator expressed as a percentage and calculated by subtracting variable operating costs from operating revenue divided by operating revenue

***Corrective action plan** specific plan with measurable goals, timelines for completion, and assigned accountability

Cost avoidance deferring a potential expense that does not have any measurable impact on the bottom line

Cost of capital required minimum return to make a project or investment worthwhile to justify its cost; often used to satisfy internal financial goals or the lowest acceptable threshold or **hurdle rate**

Cost of waste total measurable expense incurred by the business enterprise caused by clinically ineffective care and administratively inefficient processes; also **cost of poor quality**

Cost-shifting charging more to one group of patients or payers to make up for other lesser reimbursing, such as negotiating a higher rate with a commercial insurance company to make up for lower government payer reimbursement

Cost-to-charge ratio (CCR) ratio between a provider healthcare organization's expenses and what it charges payers for services

Current assets short-term or near-term assets, such as cash

Days cash on hand number of days the business enterprise could continue to pay its average daily cash obligations without any new cash resources

***Demand analysis** process to forecast patient volumes for a specified service within a certain timeframe

Demand matching formal process to determine the most appropriate physician preference item implant for each patient based on objective clinical need

Diagnosis related group (DRG) specific unique code assigned to all hospital inpatients based on their clinical diagnosis

---

* Use of this Tool or Technique is described in the book.

Direct expense costs associated with providing patient care services, such as nursing, medical supplies, drugs, and food

Discount rate rate at which future cash flows are discounted to account for time preference used to estimate how much the project's future cash flows would be worth in the present

*****Discounted cash flow analysis (DCF)** process for evaluating expected future value of cash flow from a potential project by estimating the present value of the expected future value of the cash flows it will generate

Discounting determining the present value of a future lump sum

Efficiency indicators measures amount of resources the business enterprise uses to provide services

Efficiency variance measures the impact of labor hours or supply usage on the business enterprise's financial performance; used to assess staffing effectiveness or supply utilization to meet volume demands

Exempt employee that receives a fixed salary regardless of the number of hours worked, usually with some managerial responsibilities and not entitled to overtime pay

Expense amount of money paid to provide services; also **operating expense** or **cost**

Expense budget projected annual operating costs based on forecasted service volume from the statistical budget

Fee for service reimbursement model with payment for the volume of services provided based on a fixed case rate

*****Financial condition analysis** deliberate method for reviewing and interpreting financial statements, operating indicators, and financial ratios to identify and implement opportunities for improving financial performance

Financial controls pre-established variance limits or thresholds to provide guidance for identifying and managing variances to budget targets

*****Financial modeling** process for creating as accurate a forecast as possible of a project's expected revenue and expenses

*****Financial pathway variance analysis** best practice framework and step-by-step process for analyzing a monthly profit and loss financial statement, interpreting variances, and taking the appropriate mitigating action to improve financial performance

*****Financial ratio analysis** technique to assess financial and operating performance using both financial statement and operating indicator analyses to measure profitability, liquidity, asset management, and debt management

Financial risk present whenever there is some chance of earning a return on an investment that is less than projected or required

Fiscal year (FY) annual accounting period in which financial activity is measured and reported

Fixed assets capital resources such as property, plant, and equipment

Fixed expense operating costs that do not vary with changes in volume, such as salaries, rent, and equipment depreciation

Full-time equivalent (FTE) standard unit of labor measurement typically comprised of 2,080 total paid hours when an employee works an average of 40 hours per week

Future value (FV) estimate of value of future cash flows derived from the use of an asset at some point in the future

Gross charges amount of money charged or billed for providing services; also **charges** or **gross revenue**

---

* Use of this Tool or Technique is described in the book.

Group purchasing organization (GPO) company that leverages purchasing power to negotiate discounts with manufacturers, distributers, and other vendors passed on to the business enterprise

Herfindahl-Hirschman Index (HHI) commonly accepted measure of market concentration calculated by squaring the market share of each firm competing in the service area and then summing the resulting numbers

Incidence rate calculated by dividing the number of new cases of a disease by the number of persons at risk for the disease

Income statement financial statement comparing the business enterprise's revenue and expenses to determine profitability; also **operating statement, activity statement,** or **profit and loss statement (P&L)**

Indirect expense costs associated with patient care support services typically not involving direct care such as clinical laboratory, facility maintenance, and housekeeping

Input cost indicators measure the quantity of inputs used and the cost per unit of input such as labor

Insourcing providing a product or service internal to the business enterprise

Intensity of service indicators measures the costs of providing services and the associated revenues

Interest rate (I) opportunity cost or "rent" associated with deferring the use or receipt of scarce monetary resources into the future

Internal rate of return (IRR) rate of growth a project is expected to generate and discount rate at which the present value of the costs of a project is equal to the present value of its expected revenue or the rate that produces a net present value of zero

Inventory turnover measures the dollars of total revenue generated by each dollar of inventory

Inventory turnover ratio measures a business enterprise's dollars of total revenue generated by each dollar of inventory

Investments securities the business enterprise purchases as a long-term investment such as mutual funds and bonds

Just in time (JIT) inventory designed to increase efficiency and reduce unnecessary expense by receiving products only as they are needed for use to avoid over- or understocking

Labor productivity measures how efficiently the business enterprise uses its human resources (employees) to deliver services

***Labor productivity analysis** formal process for assessing the efficiency of labor use through one or more common measures and benchmarks

Labor rate total cost for salary or wages and all benefits paid largely determined by fair market value and the supply and demand for the specific skill set

Labor ratio industry standard labor efficiency measure calculated by dividing total labor cost by total revenue

Lagging indicator financial impact resulting from implementing a quality performance improvement initiative

Leading indicator quality performance improvement measure, such as clinical outcomes or patient experience

Length of stay indicators measures business enterprise efficiency from the number of days that a patient stays in the hospital

Liabilities obligations to pay an entity with **current liabilities** typically due within 1 year and **long-term liabilities** due in more than 1 year

Liquidity ratio measures the business enterprise's ability to meet its short-term or cash obligations as they become due

---

* Use of this Tool or Technique is described in the book.

Market actual or virtual place where the business enterprise interacts with its customers directly or through intermediaries

*****Market analysis** process to define and assess the strategic challenges and opportunities for growing market share, including projected demand and the impact of competitors

Market segment sub-set of patients who share one or more common characteristics, such as geography, clinical need, or type of insurance

Market-share pricing vendor pricing model allowing increasing tiered-level discounts for physician preference items based on the amount spent

Matrix pricing vendor pricing model capping the total price a vendor can charge for each type of physician preference item regardless of the sum of individual component costs

Mode of care all clinical settings in which patients are treated, such as the outpatient clinic or intensive care unit

*****Monetizing quality** identifying the measurable financial impact from a current or proposed quality improvement initiative

*****Monthly operations review (MOR)** process to engage key stakeholders for systematically and continuously reviewing operating and financial performance variances to determine corrective actions to achieve prescribed targets

Net assets value the organization has to its owners and proportion of the assets left over after all liabilities have been paid; also **owner's equity**

Net income (or loss) amount of money remaining from net revenue after paying all expenses; also **net operating income, profit** or **(surplus)** or **loss (deficit)** if negative, and **EBITDA** (earnings before interest, taxes, depreciation, and amortization) used mostly in for-profit organizations

Net present value (NPV) sum of all the present values of the future cash flows for a project

Net revenue amount of money collected from a payer for providing services; also **net operating revenue** or **reimbursement**

Non-exempt employee compensated on an hourly basis and paid overtime usually for working more than 40 hours per week

Non-labor expense non-labor operating expense such as medical supplies, drugs, medical devices, and purchased services

Non-labor productivity measures how efficiently the business enterprise uses its non-human resources, such as supplies and purchased services

Non-productive hours paid employee hours attributed to all the non-work activities, such as paid time off or vacation, sick time, bereavement, orientation, education, and training

Occupancy rate measures inpatient volume as a percentage of the number of staffed beds; also **occupancy**

*****Open position review** process for reviewing open or vacant positions to justify filling them or to explore viable alternatives, such as job-sharing and reducing the position to part-time

Operating budget forecast of future revenue and expenses for a specific business enterprise over a period of time, such as a year

*****Operating budget** process for forecasting and providing leadership guidance on future annual volume, revenue, and expenses

*****Operating indicator analysis** assess financial and operating performance using specific data primarily from the business enterprise's managerial accounting system to measure profitability, price, volume, length of stay, intensity of service, efficiency, and input cost

Operating indicators measures business enterprise financial condition including profitability, price, volume, length of stay, intensity of service, efficiency, and input cost

---

* Use of this Tool or Technique is described in the book.

Operating margin key financial performance indicator measuring the amount of operating profit per dollar of operating expense expressed as a percentage and calculated by subtracting operating costs from operating revenues divided by operating revenue; also **margin**

Opportunity cost financial benefit given up from using an existing resource for another purpose

Outsourcing contracting with an external vendor or supplier to provide a service to improve quality performance or reduce cost

Overhead expense fixed cost not associated with volume including management and support to run the organization such as executive salaries, human resources, marketing, and legal fees; also **overhead** or **fully loaded expense**

Paid hours total hours the employee is paid categorized as productive or non-productive

Par level lowest stock volume that can be maintained without risking running short yet low enough to avoid over-stocking

Patient responsibility portion of the total payment for service owed by the patient after any insurance coverage payment including a deductible or co-pay; also **patient obligation** or **patient burden**

Payback period length of time it takes to recover the initial investment in a project without considering the time value of money

Payer entity responsible for paying for services, such as Medicare, private insurance, an employer, or individual; also **payor**

Pay-for-performance (P4P) payment to achieve a specific performance measure

Physician preference items (PPI) typically high-cost implantable medical devices, such as cardiac defibrillators and orthopedic hip and knee prosthetics

Population health management holistic approach to improving health outcomes for a specific group as part of the movement toward value-based care

Present value (PV) estimate of current value of future cash flows derived from an initiative or investment based on making reasonable projections of how much revenue it will generate

Prevalence rate total number of cases of a disease existing in a population divided by the total population

Price indicators measure a market's assessment of the value of the services provided by the business enterprise

Primary service area (PSA) geographic zone defined by the zip codes, usually contiguous or connecting, that comprises 75 to 80 percent of its patients based on where they live

Pro forma statement with projected financial performance based on expectations about anticipated volume, revenue, and expenses

*Process mapping defining a specific process through direct observation to identify all steps and activities to assess problems or common areas of inefficiency; also **flow charting**

Process of care all the functions and systems for delivering services, such as scheduling, registration, and care delivery

Productive hours paid employee hours attributed to all work activities including breaks and lunch

Profit per discharge (or clinic visit) measures the amount of profit or the contribution to net income earned on each unit of service calculated by subtracting operating expenses from operating revenue divided by total volume

*Profitability analysis basic assessment of a business enterprise's financial performance or profitability calculated by subtracting operating expense from operating revenue to determine the net income

---

* Use of this Tool or Technique is described in the book.

Profitability ratios measure business enterprise operating profitability, such as profit per inpatient discharge and profit per outpatient visit

*****Rapid cycle testing (RCT)** implement a small test of change and observe the impact to proof the concept prior to a potentially time-consuming and costly full implementation; also **pilot**

Rate variance measures the impact of the labor cost (or rate) or supply price on the business enterprise's financial performance

Request for proposal (RFP) formal process to invite competitive pricing bids from qualified vendors

Resource-based costing a holistic way to estimate costs for a proposed project

Return on investment (ROI) measures financial performance of an investment reported in dollar terms or rate of return

Revenue budget projected annual gross and net revenues based on forecasted service volume from the statistical budget

Revenue cycle how money typically flows through a healthcare provider organization from billing through collections

*****Risk analysis** process to objectively identify and evaluate potential risks for doing a project or not doing a project and how to disengage if the project is unsuccessful

Seasonality changes in volume, revenue, and expenses due to predictable market or environmental factors, such as flu season

Secondary service area (SSA) geographic zone defined by the zip codes, usually contiguous or connecting, that comprises 20% to 25% of its patients based on where they live

*****Secret shopping** interacting with competitors to understand if and how the business enterprise is meeting its customers' needs to improve competitive differentiation

*****Sensitivity analysis** project analysis technique to assess how changes in a single input variable, such as volume affects profitability

Service recovery actions taken typically as part of a formal program to convert customer issues to increase brand loyalty

Shared savings incentive payment typically paid to providers for reducing expense without compromising established quality standards; also gain sharing

Skill mix blend of technical or clinical skill used to deliver service ideally with all employees working at the top of their license

*****Span of control analysis** process for assessing opportunities to flatten the management structure to improve decision-making efficiency and reduce unnecessary labor expense

*****Staffing to demand** alternative to traditional shift staffing by varying or flexing staff according to volume demands

Standard order set clinical order for a specific medical condition or procedure intended to hardwire best practice care and reduce unwarranted clinical variation

Statement of cash flows financial statement showing the business enterprise's cash resources including where they came from and how they were used during the accounting period to determine if the organization can generate enough cash to meet both short- and long-term obligations

Statistical budget projected service volume typically based on historical data and any market changes used to develop the revenue and expense budgets

Time value of money a dollar in hand today is worth more than a dollar that will be received at some point in the future due to inflation and the ability to invest it

Timeline visual representation of the time horizon within which all relevant asset cash flows are presumed to occur

---

* Use of this Tool or Technique is described in the book.

Total asset turnover ratio measures business enterprise's dollars of total revenue per dollar of total assets

Total margin measures profitability as a percentage of total revenues and the business enterprise's ability to control expenses calculated by subtracting total costs from total revenues divided by total revenue

Trend analysis used to assess changes in key financial and operating indicators, both favorable and unfavorable, over a period of time

Unit of service (UoS) standard patient volume activity statistic used for variance and other calculations, such as an admission, clinic visit, or surgical procedure

Value quality divided by cost, inextricably linked variables

Value analysis process (VAP) formal process to engage key clinical, operational, and financial stakeholders and end-users typically through a service-line specific value analysis team

Value analysis team (VAT) empowered to assess and select or recommend products and services that optimize quality, safety, and cost

Value-based care reimbursement model with payment for achieving specified outcomes

Value proposition an innovation, service, or feature that makes a product or service attractive to customers

Variable expense operating costs that change based on patient volume, such as scheduled hourly labor and supplies

Variance difference between the operating or financial targets of the business enterprise and actual performance that can be favorable or unfavorable

Variance analysis deliberate and systematic process for identifying the root cause or causes of the difference between operating or financial targets and actual performance

Volume indicators measure business enterprise patient activity, typically related to profitability

Volume variance measures impact of patient volume on the business enterprise's financial performance

Waste anything that does not support improving value

Weighted cost of capital (WACC) proportionately weighted cost of acquiring money from different sources such as stock and bonds

---

* Use of this Tool or Technique is described in the book.

APPENDICES

Appendix A: Regional Health System Case Example: Background

Regional Health System (RHS) is an integrated health system serving a total population of approximately 350,000 people. It is a not-for-profit, community-based health system that provides a full range of inpatient, out-patient, emergency, urgent, and post-acute care services to the residents of the service area in which it operates. RHS operates an acute care hospital, critical access hospital, skilled nursing facility, and a dozen freestanding outpatient treatment facilities, including primary and multi-specialty care clinics, retail clinics, and an ambulatory surgery center. RHS consists of the following healthcare provider organizations:

- Regional Medical Center (RMC): 300 beds (staffed)
- Regional Community Hospital (RCH): 25 beds (staffed)
- Regional Nursing Center (RCN): 50 beds (skilled nursing)

A summary of the consolidated financials provided in Appendix B show that RHS has increasing gross revenue in the 3-year period from 20XX to 20X2; however, decreasing net income due to increasing operating expenses is outstripping revenue.

	12/31/20XX	12/31/20X1	12/31/20X2
Total Operating Revenue	$204,043,674	$206,395,461	$210,934,576
Total Operating Expenses	$186,667,981	$192,262,218	$202,630,146
Net Income	$17,375,693	$14,133,243	$8,304,430

Due to continued financial challenges straining already thin operating margins the CEO has implemented austerity measures to examine and control costs wherever possible.

Appendix B: Consolidated Financial Statements and Selected Measures of Financial and Operating Performance for Regional Health System, FY 20XX to FY 20X2

FINANCIAL STATEMENTS			
INCOME STATEMENT	**12/31/20XX**	**12/31/20X1**	**12/31/20X2**	**PEER GROUP AVERAGE**
Inpatient Revenue	$253,327,486	$272,999,473	$295,211,498	$182,227,234
Outpatient Revenue	$283,779,957	$312,904,961	$349,532,119	$182,975,949
Gross Revenue	$537,107,443	$585,904,434	$644,743,617	$349,955,188
Allowances & Discounts	$334,917,193	$381,150,008	$435,795,336	$238,519,161
Net Patient Revenue	$202,190,250	$204,754,426	$208,948,281	$110,016,270
Other Nonpatient Revenue	$1,853,424	$1,641,035	$1,986,295	$4,955,059
Total Operating Revenue	$204,043,674	$206,395,461	$210,934,576	$114,320,345
Depreciation Expense	$15,482,870	$11,984,457	$13,318,450	$5,662,550
Other Expenses	$171,185,111	$180,277,761	$189,311,696	$101,730,314
Total Operating Expenses	$186,667,981	$192,262,218	$202,630,146	$108,661,972
Net Income	$17,375,693	$14,133,243	$8,304,430	$5,658,374
BALANCE SHEET	**12/31/20XX**	**12/31/20X1**	**12/31/20X2**	**PEER GROUP AVERAGE**
Cash	$1,554,517	$895,275	$2,461,730	$14,550,593
Accounts Receivable	$38,151,068	$31,777,990	$31,328,655	$19,243,350
Other Current Assets	$2,299,210	$2,230,485	$3,687,531	$19,785,315
Total Current Assets	$42,004,795	$34,903,750	$37,477,916	$54,607,042
Gross Fixed Assets	$205,784,933	$218,120,890	$226,384,012	$111,011,445
Accumulated Depreciation	$102,986,899	$114,466,564	$126,860,189	$63,201,406
Net Fixed Assets	$102,798,034	$103,654,326	$99,523,823	$57,644,244
Investments	$202,907,104	$212,569,850	$0	$12,589,537
Other Assets	$0	$0	$244,101,733	$20,223,644
Total Assets	$347,709,933	$351,127,926	$381,103,472	$144,677,432
Current Liabilities	$70,267,452	$54,354,094	$57,433,940	$21,851,240
Long-Term Liabilities	$78,969,672	$75,939,927	$81,950,624	$41,134,926
Total Liabilities	$149,237,124	$130,294,021	$139,384,564	$65,030,137
Fund Balance	$198,472,809	$220,833,905	$231,866,348	$80,859,987
Total Liabilities and Fund Balance	$347,709,933	$351,127,926	$371,250,912	$144,700,548

RATIO ANALYSIS				
PROFITABILITY INDICATORS	12/31/20XX	12/31/20X1	12/31/20X2	PEER GROUP AVERAGE
Total Margin	11.7	9.4	20.2	-4.8
Operating Margin	8.2	6.7	3.3	-5.6
Nonoperating Margin	3.5	2.7	17.0	0.8
Deductible Ratio	62.4	65.1	67.6	59.5
Markup Ratio	2.9	3.1	3.2	2.9
Return on Total Assets	7.1	5.6	13.5	7.9
Return on Equity	12.4	9.0	21.3	14.2
Return on Investment	0.2	0.1	0.3	0.1
LIQUIDITY RATIOS				
Current Ratio	0.6	0.6	0.7	3.3
Average Payment Period	149.8	110.0	110.7	79.7
Days Cash on Hand	3.3	1.8	4.7	26.3
Days in Accounts Receivable	68.9	56.6	54.7	62.9
ASSET EFFICIENCY RATIOS				
Total Asset Turnover	0.61	0.60	0.67	1.42
Fixed Asset Turnover	2.06	2.05	2.55	8.23
Current Asset Turnover	5.03	6.08	6.78	3.11
Net Fixed Assets per Bed	204,577	203,786	192,276	132,415
Average Age of Plant	6.7	9.6	9.5	18.9
OPERATING INDICATOR ANALYSIS				
PROFITABILITY INDICATORS	12/31/20XX	12/31/20X1	12/31/20X2	PEER GROUP AVERAGE
Profit per Discharge	$511	$395	$172	$216
Profit per Outpatient Visit	$36	$33	$31	$29
PRICE INDICATORS				
Gross Price per Discharge	$17,665	$18,523	$17,556	$35,737
Net Price per Discharge	$6,650	$6,473	$5,690	$12,724
VOLUME INDICATORS				
Hospital Beds	237	237	237	121
Discharges	13,998	14,320	16,294	15,274
Births	2,104	2,183	2,134	2,536
Patient Days	62,298	64,817	62,898	25,725
Average Daily Census (Hospital)	177.5	170.6	164.2	168.6

Occupancy (Hospital)	72.0	74.9	72.5	50.5
Outpatient Visits	33,977	45,073	53,127	42,961
Emergency Department Visits	80,832	82,240	82,444	92,347
Surgeries and Endoscopies	17,055	16,332	16,168	26,297
LENGTH OF STAY INDICATORS				
Length of Stay	4.5	4.5	3.9	8.2
Length of Stay (CMA)	3.1	3.2	2.9	3.0
INTENSITY OF SERVICE INDICATORS				
Case Mix Index (CMI)	1.4241	1.4045	1.3410	1.4089
INPUT COST INDICATORS				
Cost per Discharge	$6,139	$6,078	$5,518	$13,503
Cost per Discharge (CMA, WIA)	$4,366	$4,707	$4,504	$6,733
Salaries per Discharge	$2,526	$2,606	$2,266	$5,349
Salaries per Discharge (CMA, WIA)	$1,797	$2,018	$1,850	$2,523
Capital Costs per Discharge	$509	$379	$363	$605
Capital Costs per Discharge (CMA, WIA)	$362	$293	$296	$404
General Service Cost per Discharge	$2,535	$2,630	$2,508	$4,993
General Service Cost per Discharge (CMA, WIA)	$1,803	$2,037	$2,047	$2,650
FTEs per Occupied Bed	4.26	4.44	4.56	5.14
FTEs per Occupied Bed (CMA)	2.99	3.16	3.40	4.06
Paid Hours per Discharge	108	114	100	226
Paid Hours per Discharge (CMA)	75.90	81.45	74.77	91.73
Facility Salary per FTE	$48,618	$47,376	$47,015	$51,321
Facility Salary per FTE (WIA)	$49,243	$51,529	$51,467	$59,324
Facility Wage Index	0.9873	0.9194	0.9135	0.8896
PAYER MIX				
Outpatient Revenue Percentage	52.8	53.4	54.2	54.2
Inpatient Revenue Percentage	47.2	46.6	45.8	50.3

Appendix C: Financial Pathway for Department of Surgical Services at Regional Health System

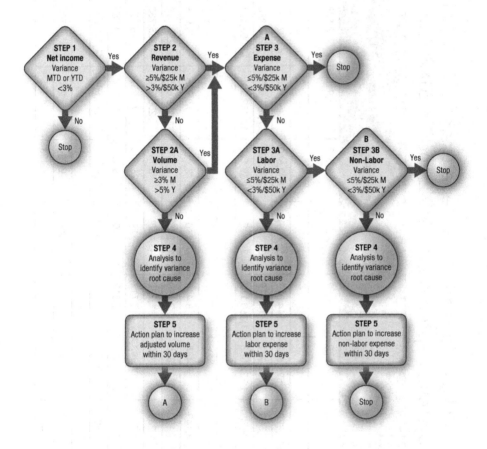

M, month; MTD, month-to-date; Y, year; YTD, year-to-date.

Appendix D: Profit and Loss Statement for Department of Surgical Services at Regional Health System, September FY 20X2 and FY 20X2 Year-to-Date

	SEPTEMBER (FY 20X2)				FY 20X2 YEAR-TO-DATE			
	PRIOR YEAR ACTUAL	BUDGET	ACTUAL	VARIANCE	PRIOR YEAR ACTUAL	BUDGET	ACTUAL	VARIANCE
Total Units of Service (Adjusted Surgeries)	712	670	699	29	2,038	1,916	2,528	612
OPERATING REVENUE								
Total Inpatient Revenue	610,220	599,662	544,053	(55,609)	1,830,660	4,860,920	4,802,591	(58,329)
Total Outpatient Revenue	769,500	732,921	816,079	83,158	2,308,500	7,291,381	7,203,886	(87,495)
Total Operating Revenue	1,379,720	1,332,583	1,360,132	27,549	4,139,160	12,152,301	12,006,477	(145,824)
OPERATING EXPENSES								
Labor Expenses								
3010 Director Salary	8,149	8,444	8,444	0	73,215	75,996	75,996	0
3020 RN Salaries & Wages	172,190	131,845	172,190	(40,345)	516,570	1,186,605	1,253,328	(66,723)
3030 LVN Salaries & Wages	31,238	27,800	31,238	(3,438)	93,714	250,200	265,788	(15,588)
3050 Aide Salaries & Wages	8,712	7,993	8,712	(719)	26,136	71,937	76,331	(4,394)
3070 Clerical Salaries & Wages	3,312	3,312	3,312	0	10,959	29,808	28,855	953
Total Labor Expenses	223,601	179,394	223,896	(44,502)	720,594	1,614,546	1,700,298	(85,752)
Non-Labor Expenses								
5010 Continuing Medical Education	0	246	0	246	2,134	2,214	1,500	714
7000 Office Supplies	444	485	417	68	5,433	4,365	4,211	154

	SEPTEMBER (FY 20X2)				FY 20X2 YEAR-TO-DATE			
	PRIOR YEAR ACTUAL	BUDGET	ACTUAL	VARIANCE	PRIOR YEAR ACTUAL	BUDGET	ACTUAL	VARIANCE
7010 Minor Equipment	2,566	2,705	2,433	272	22,877	24,345	25,443	(1,098)
7030 Med/Surg Supplies	59,778	63,043	80,125	(17,082)	543,778	567,387	599,987	(32,600)
7080 IV Supplies	2,026	1,927	2,185	(258)	14,567	17,343	19,552	(2,209)
7110 Lithrotripsy Fee	3,025	2,459	2,100	359	18,998	22,131	20,047	2,084
7130 Pacers	11,915	18,448	13,960	4,488	156,332	166,032	164,687	1,345
7150 Sutures	2,063	3,279	4,991	(1,712)	26,880	29,511	30,558	(1,047)
7200 Orthopedic Implants	143,675	124,789	142,436	(17,647)	986,334	1,123,101	1,183,420	(60,319)
7300 Instrument Repair/Replace	3,168	6,969	5,256	1,713	57,990	62,721	58,574	4,147
7310 Staples	9,849	10,659	11,525	(866)	90,447	95,931	101,154	(5,223)
7320 Drug Supply Expense	37	394	2,307	(1,913)	3,222	3,546	5,438	(1,892)
7500 Linens & Scrubs	135	1,254	1,894	(640)	9,008	11,286	11,041	245
7600 Repairs & Maintenance	0	1,468	1,312	156	15,442	13,212	12,650	562
7850 Other Contract Services	(12,243)	14,415	4,117	10,298	118,065	129,735	127,443	2,292
Total Non-Labor Expenses	226,438	252,540	275,058	(22,518)	2,071,507	2,272,860	2,365,705	(92,845)
Total Operating Expense	450,039	431,934	498,954	(67,020)	2,792,101	3,887,406	4,066,003	(178,597)
Net Income/(Loss)	929,681	900,649	861,178	(39,471)	1,347,059	8,264,895	7,940,474	(324,421)

Appendix E: Thirty Proven Tactics to Optimize Labor Productivity

1. Eliminate use of premium labor (e.g., contract, agency)

2. Reduce overtime—incidental, scheduled, and other (no more than 3% of total compensation)

3. Evaluate on-call need; consider utilization and alternatives

4. Minimize non-variable (fixed) staff

5. Evaluate orientation and education needs and programs

6. Use non-traditional shifts and flexing

7. Share staff with other departments

8. Float staff to similar units

9. Consider day of week adjustments

10. Consolidate positions, cross-train as needed

11. Establish sister units for demand or overflow

12. Consolidate units/functions (temporary or permanent)

13. Change skill mix to achieve "top of license" optimization (e.g., LPN vs RN)

14. Create flexible core staff versus only full-time—evaluate use of part-time and per diem

15. Do schedulable work during predictable slow periods (e.g., patient callbacks, inventory, paperwork)

16. Delay non-critical work to slower day, week, or period

17. Change hours of operation (e.g., close earlier)

18. Improve the process—apply Lean-Six Sigma change concepts to eliminate non-value-added work

19. Implement revised staffing plan based on identified opportunities

20. Adjust staffing every 2 hours (or 4 hours) versus every 8 hours

21. During a slow period requiring minimum staffing, take on work from another department so it can reduce worked hours

22. Fill overflow work by finding a department with capacity versus using overtime

23. Rather than fill open positions, identify another department with a vacancy and merge positions into one job

24. Rather than fill an open position, reduce to less hours (part-time)

25. Absorb additional volume during short duration volume increases—"stretch"

26. Stagger lunch, dinner, and other breaks

27. Pre-plan vacations/time off to predictably slower periods versus as requested by staff

28. Offer variable shifts to older workers, new parents

29. Decrease management layers, increase span of control, and decrease supervisory hours

30. Smooth or shape incoming demand to earlier or later in the day to better match staffing pattern

Appendix F: Purchased Services Inventory Checklist

1. SUPPORT SERVICES		
☐ Food service	☐ Environmental services	☐ Biomedical maintenance
☐ Linen (laundry and uniforms)	☐ Waste/recycling (regular)	☐ Waste (medical)
☐ Landscaping	☐ Pest control	☐ Medical gasses
☐ Fire/safety inspection	☐ Clinical engineering/ biomed maintenance	☐ Other _____
2. CLINICAL AND ANCILLARY SERVICES		
☐ Reference lab	☐ Pharmacy	☐ 340B Pharmacy program
☐ Therapy (PT, OT, speech)	☐ Blood bank	☐ Dialysis
☐ Wound care	☐ Diagnostic imaging interpretation	☐ Other _____
3. INFORMATION SYSTEMS AND TECHNOLOGY		
☐ Office automation (copiers, fax, scanner, printers)	☐ Telephone service (local/ long distance, cellular and paging)	☐ Conference calling
☐ Call center	☐ Answering service	☐ Postage machines
☐ Computer purchasing and support	☐ Quick copy services	☐ Other_____
4. HEALTH MANAGEMENT INFORMATION SERVICES		
☐ Charts and records processing	☐ Document management (storage, shredding)	☐ Courier (document/ specimen)
☐ Transcription services	☐ Electronic health record (EHR)	☐ Overnight delivery
5. SUPPLIES		
☐ Office supplies and furniture	☐ Medical supplies	☐ Oncology supplies
☐ X-ray supplies/services	☐ Pharmaceuticals	☐ Vaccines
6. HUMAN RESOURCES		
☐ Employment screening	☐ Wealth management 401(k) and financial planning	☐ Statement processing
☐ Agency (clinical/admin)	☐ Other_____	
7. REVENUE CYCLE		
☐ Banking	☐ Claims processing	☐ Payroll processing
☐ Credit card processing	☐ Collection services	☐ Other _____
8. MARKETING		
☐ Advertising promotional	☐ Forms and printing	☐ Advertising (Yellow Pages)

9. MEDICAL STAFF		
☐ Provider recruiting	☐ Medical publications	☐ Insurance
☐ Magazine subscriptions	☐ Other _____	
10. OTHER		
☐ Real estate/building management	☐ Other _____	

Appendix G: Secret Shopping Script (Orthopedic Clinic Example)

Secret Shopper: Hi, my name is _____ and we recently moved here from out-of-state. We're looking to schedule an appointment for our 4-year-old son. Do you have openings?

Clinic: *What happens to be bothering him?*

Secret Shopper: He's been walking a little funny lately. He favors his right leg when he walks. We saw our family doc just before we left Minnesota and she suggested we get him looked at by an orthopedic specialist. It's not urgent but I would like to get him in as soon as we can to get it figured out.

Clinic: *Asks for more detail on injury, history, and treatment.*

Secret Shopper: Started noticing limp a couple weeks ago. No apparent injury. Does not complain of pain but right foot sensitive to touch. Doesn't have trouble sleeping. Has not limited his activities. No x-rays or MRIs have been done.
No health issues in the past.

Clinic: *What type of insurance do you have?*

Secret Shopper: We have _____ (specify common commercial insurance plan in market).

Clinic: *Do you have your insurance information on hand?*

Secret Shopper: No, I actually don't have it on me right now, sorry.

Clinic: *That's fine. Please have it when you come in. We can get you in this Wednesday at 3 pm. Does that work for you?*

Secret Shopper: Sorry, that time won't work. When is the next available? Also, would this appointment be with a provider?

Clinic: *Yes, with Dr. Reed, a pediatric orthopedist. How about Thursday at 4?*

Secret Shopper: We will be out of town then. Is there another time after that?

Clinic: *I have Monday the 19th at 2 o'clock.*

Secret Shopper: That may work. Let me check with my spouse and I will call you back if the time works. Just out of curiosity, do you offer after-hours evening or weekend appointments? *(if so, how late and on what days)*?

Appendix H: Provider Liaison Qualifications

The Provider Liaison can be an effective role to support the business enterprise's provider relations and market share growth goals. A high level of professionalism and respect in all interactions is the most important attribute, however successful incumbents typically come from clinical or sales backgrounds. Each background has distinct advantages listed in Table H1.

TABLE H1 Provider Liaison Background Advantages

CLINICAL ADVANTAGE	SALES ADVANTAGE
• Credibility with providers • Not regarded as a sales person • Accurate communication of patient diagnosis, problems, and needs, effectively responding to provider questions • Clinical knowledge to address provider concerns • Deeper access and insight into clinical rumor mill for sales intelligence • Working knowledge of providers' motivations • Provider relations experience	• Experience and comfort with goal management • Revenue oriented • Persistence and follow-through • Ability to close deals • Negotiating skills • Strategic alignment of product (hospital services) with provider need • Probes for below-surface insight and intelligence • Confidence in asking for business • Persuasive presentation skills

Regardless of the background and experience, interpersonal skills weigh more heavily than clinical or sales experience. Consider using a personality assessment test to learn more detail about each candidate's behavioral tendencies, the most desirable of which are listed in Table H2.

TABLE H2 Desirable Behavioral Traits of the Provider Liaison

• Relationship-driven • Exceptional communication skills • Extroverted and enthusiastic • Confident • Entrepreneurial • Self-motivated and driven • Conscientious work habits • Industrious • Positive, can-do attitude	• Goal-oriented • Negotiating skills • Persuasive and influential • Customer service-oriented • Creative • Action oriented • Excellent follow-through • Accountability • Organized and thorough • Critical thinking and problem-solving

The Provider Liaison must be able to communicate effectively with a broad spectrum of healthcare provider organization staff—from CEOs to surgeons to receptionists—and should be prepared to spend the large majority of their time outside the office. When evaluating candidates' employment references it is important to explore their integrity, expertise, flexibility, and perseverance.

Appendix I: Provider Alignment Survey

I. Scale

A. Strongly Agree

B. Agree

C. Neither Agree nor Disagree

D. Disagree

E. Strongly Disagree

II. Survey Domains, Operational Definitions, and Questions

A *Rulemaking.* Instituting evidence-based best practices through required use of organization-provided tools and processes; such as electronic medical record, standard order set, and drug formulary.

1. Providers are involved in establishing evidence-based clinical practice guidelines.

2. Evidence-based clinical practice guidelines are clearly communicated to providers.

3. Evidence-based clinical practice guidelines are adhered to by providers.

4. Providers are involved in the periodic review of peer clinical outcomes compared to evidence-based practice guidelines.

B. *Communicating Performance.* Providers are given accurate, timely, and actionable data, information, and feedback; such as an organizational dashboard, individual scorecard, and financial reports with comparative internal/peer benchmarks.

5. Strategic goals are clearly communicated throughout the organization.

6. Performance expectations regarding desired clinical outcomes are communicated to providers.

7. Providers are given actionable clinical data to improve outcomes.

8. Performance expectations regarding desired financial goals are communicated to providers.

9. Providers are given actionable financial data to improve financial performance.

10. Providers clinical outcomes are benchmarked against internal/peer best practices.

C. *Supported Change.* Offering providers organization-sponsored "how to" instruction, training and education and ongoing coaching and mentoring to achieve best practices.

11. The organization provides ongoing professional development for providers to improve clinical outcomes.

12. The organization provides ongoing professional development for providers to improve their business/financial acumen.

13. Providers are offered ongoing support to address identified gaps in achieving best practice.

14. Providers are surveyed periodically to provide their input for ways to improve organizational performance.

15. Organizational leaders support providers' delivering the best possible care for their patients.

D. *Governance and Leadership.* Installing and cultivating formal provider leaders throughout all levels of the organization (e.g., board, c-suite, department) to set and achieve strategic goals and to participate in key financial and operational improvement venues (e.g., budgeting, clinical service lines, value analysis).

16. Providers participate broadly in developing organizational strategy.

17. Provider and administrative leaders share decision-making authority across all levels of the organization.

18. Providers are involved in setting and achieving financial and operating goals (e.g., annual budget and capital spending).

19. Providers are involved in data governance to improve decision-making efficacy, such as how data are collected, validated, and reported.

20. Providers are involved in selecting vendors that provide supplies and service.

E. *Structural Framework.* Creating formal organization-sponsored relationships with providers that enable their participation in compliant risk/reward models, such as employment, joint venture, management services organization, providers-hospital organization, co-management.

21. Leadership supports mutually beneficial partnership arrangements with providers that align their interests with organizational goals, such as joint ventures.

22. Organization sponsors formal models that support providers' practice needs, such as provider-hospital organization, management services organization, and independent practice association.

23. Collaborative structures equally engage all members of the medical staff, both employed and independent providers, to support achieving organizational goals.

24. Work teams comprised of providers and staff are empowered by leadership to make changes to improve organizational performance.

25. Providers participate in value-based reimbursement models that support improving clinical outcomes, such as bundled payments, accountable care organization, patient-centered medical home.

F. *Risk and Reward.* Offering "skin in the game" pay-for-performance bonuses and/or risk-based penalties based on achieving specified providers-driven goals.

26. Total providers compensation is tied to achieving organizational goals.

27. Providers are eligible to earn performance incentive compensation (e.g., bonus) for achieving specified goals.

28. Providers have some part of their total compensation "at-risk" (e.g., penalty) for failing to achieve specified goals.

29. Providers are involved in the process for determining pay-for-performance measures.

G. *Sociological/Cultural.* Creating an organizational culture that fosters trust, collaboration, and intrinsic motivation to achieve the organization's goals.

30. The organizational culture for setting strategic goals is largely top-down driven.

31. Providers have a sense of ownership in achieving organizational goals.

32. Providers and administrators are empowered to make changes that support organizational goals.

33. There is a high degree of trust between providers and administrators.

34. There is a high degree of collaboration between providers and administrators.

Appendix J. Basic Introduction to Electronic Spreadsheets With Video Tutorials*

The electronic spreadsheet is a powerful tool with which leaders should have a basic command of the common functions for conducting various analyses. The main benefit of electronic spreadsheets is the ease with which an analysis can be run and then rerun using a different set of assumptions. One or more variables can easily be changed to view the impact allowing leaders to conduct "what if" analyses by evaluating a wide range of assumptions.

Performing advanced calculations, such as net present value and internal rate of return, will be presented later in the appendix. A basic overview will provide those new to electronic spreadsheets a working knowledge. In addition, there are extensive free online resources and tutorials, some of which are listed in the References. Specific configurations and settings will vary based on the software version and the operating system (PC and Mac).

Creating a New Electronic Spreadsheet

Creating a new spreadsheet can be done by selecting File then Open or New Document in the top toolbar menu as shown in Figure J.1.

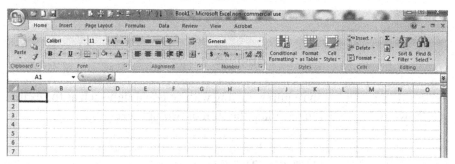

FIGURE J.1 Creating a new electronic spreadsheet.

Note the horizontal rows identified by numbers and the vertical columns identified by letters shown in Figure J.2.

---

* Video content for Appendix J is available on Springer Connect at connect.springerpub.com/content/book/ 978-0-8261-4464-5/back-matter/bmatter10.

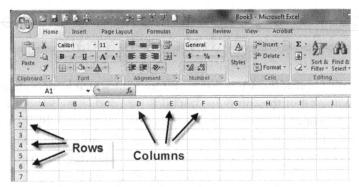

FIGURE J.2 Rows and columns.

Each individual cell such as C4 shown in Figure J.3 is the intersection of a row and column into which data can be entered including numbers, text, and formulae to perform various calculations.

	A	B	C	D	E
1					
2	CELL: C4				
3					
4					
5					
6					
7					

FIGURE J.3 Cells.

Performing a calculation requires starting with an equal sign such as the example shown in Figure J.4 to calculate the sum of two numbers.

	A	B	C
1	=128.92+347.58		
2			
3			
4			

FIGURE J.4 Entering a simple formula (adding two numbers).

After hitting the return or enter key the result or answer from the formula entered in the formula bar is automatically calculated as shown in Figure J.5.

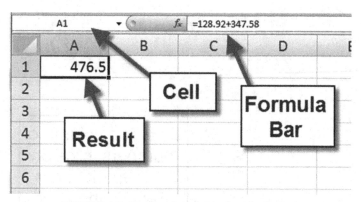

FIGURE J.5 Performing a simple calculation.

Math Operations

When entering a formula the basic math signs apply: + to add, - to subtract, * asterisk to multiply, and forward slash (/) to divide. As mentioned earlier formulae will always begin with an equal sign.

Group Numbers

It is important to understand that there is an order by which calculations are performed. Excel multiplies and divides first and then adds and subtracts second. For example, using the formula =128.92 + 347.58/3 the first operation will be dividing 347.58 by 3 and then adding 128.92. If the desired operation is to add 128.92 and 347.58 and then divide that result by 3 then a parentheses must be used as follows:

=(128.92+347.58)/3.

Functions

Excel offers a number of useful functions that provide the mathematical formulae for common and complex calculations from very simple to complex. For example, one of the most common and useful functions is the Sum function. The sum function can be used to add a column of numbers by entering =sum(number1, number2, number3...) or by using the sigma (Σ) symbol shown in Figure J.6.

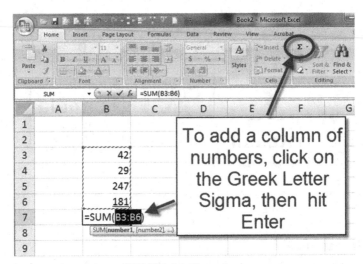

FIGURE J.6 Summing.

Other Excel functions are useful and expedient for various financial calculations such as present value (PV), net present value (NPV), and internal rate of return (IRR). Setting up a data table with the required variables will be useful for performing the calculations. The Excel variable terms and abbreviations used to calculate present value are presented in Figure J.7.

Future Value

Future value (FV) is an estimate of value of the cash flows derived from the use of an asset at some point. ⊙ See the video content at connect.springerpub.com/content/book/978-0-8261-4464-5/back-matter/bmatter10 for a brief recorded tutorial of how to calculate FV.

	A	B	C	D
1	Excel	Formula	Meaning	Data
2	rate	I	interest rate	0.1
3	nper	N	number of periods	3
4	pmt		payment	
5	pv	PV	present value	-100
6	type	0 or 1	payment at end (0) or beginning (1) of period	0

FIGURE J.7 Terms for calculating future value (FV).

Entering "FV" into a blank cell where the calculation is to be shown preceded by an equal sign provides the prompts to enter the required variables created in the data table in the previous figure as shown in Figure J.8.

	A	B	C	D	E	F
1	Excel	Formula	Meaning	Data		
2	rate	I	interest rate	0.1		
3	nper	N	number of periods	3		
4	pmt		payment			
5	pv	PV	present value	-100		
6	type	0 or 1	payment at end (0) or beginning (1) of period	0		
7						
8						
9	fv	FV	future value	=FV()		
10				FV(rate, nper, pmt, [pv], [type])		
11						

FIGURE J.8 Setting up the calculation for future value.

In this lump sum cash outflow example there is no need to enter anything for the payment (pmt). A zero or a comma will suffice. Nothing is required for the type if the payment is to be at the end of the period since this is how it calculates automatically. Assuming all of the cell references are entered correctly and displayed in the function bar window (*fx*) at the top right of this screen shot, including entering commas after each entry, the correct value of $133.10 should be displayed as shown in Figure J.9.

D9		fx	=FV(D2,D3,0,D5)	
	A	B	C	D
1	Excel	Formula	Meaning	Data
2	rate	I	interest rate	0.1
3	nper	N	number of periods	3
4	pmt		payment	
5	pv	PV	present value	-100
6	type	0 or 1	payment at end (0) or beginning (1) of period	0
7				
8				
9	fv	FV	future value	$133.10
10				

FIGURE J.9 Calculating future value.

Solving now for the present value using the Excel formula where the future value is $100 (entered as a negative number) the answer is $75.13 as shown in Figure J.10.

Present Value

Present value (PV) is an estimate of current value of future cash flows derived from an initiative or investment based on making reasonable projections of how much revenue it will generate. ⏵ See the video content at connect .springerpub.com/content/book/978-0-8261-4464-5/back-matter/bmatter10 for a brief recorded tutorial of how to calculate PV.

FIGURE J.10 Calculating present value.

Net Present Value

Net present value (NPV) is calculated using a discount rate, which may represent an interest rate or the rate of inflation, and a series of future payments (negative values) and income (positive values). ⊙ See the video content at connect .springerpub.com/content/book/978-0-8261-4464-5/back-matter/bmatter10 for a brief recorded tutorial of how to calculate NPV.

After entering the required equal sign and then "NPV" the interest rate in the data table (cell C2) can be populated in the formula window. After entering a comma the cash flows (CF) from Year 1 through Year 4 are selected by holding the shift key and move the cursor down to select the entire series as shown in Figure J.11.

FIGURE J.11 Setting up the calculation for net present value.

After entering return or enter the result for the NPV of the uneven cash flow stream for Years 1 through 4 is $530.09 as shown in Figure J.12.

C9		fx	=NPV(C2,C4:C7)		

	A	B	C	D	E
1	**Excel**	**Formula**	**Data**		
2	rate	I	0.1		
3	cash flows	CF			
4			Year 1 $ 100		
5			Year 2 $ 300		
6			Year 3 $ 300		
7			Year 4 $ (50)		
8					
9	net present value	NPV	$530.09		
10					

FIGURE J.12 Calculating NPV.

Solving another net present value problem with an initial investment or cash outflow of $1.5 million entered as a negative number with parentheses in Year 0, set up the data table with the interest rate (I) and cash flows. However, when entering the cells to calculate NPV the cash outflow in Year 0 is not included. This amount will be added to the formula after selecting the cash flow series from Years 1 through 4 as shown in the formula box in Figure J.13.

NPV		fx	=NPV(C2,C5:C8+C4)		

	A	B	C	D	E
1	**Excel**	**Formula**	**Data**		
2	rate	I	0.08		
3	cash flows	CF			
4			Year 0 $ (1,500)		
5			Year 1 $ 310		
6			Year 2 $ 400		
7			Year 3 $ 500		
8			Year 4 $ 750		
9					
10	net present value	NPV	=NPV(C2,C5:C8+C4)		
11			NPV(rate, value1, [value2], [value3], ...)		
12					

FIGURE J.13 Setting up the calculation for NPV with an initial investment in Year 0.

The calculated NPV should be $78.16 as presented in Figure J.14.

C10 | fx =NPV(C2,C5:C8)+C4

Excel	Formula	Data
rate	I	0.08
cash flows	CF	
	Year 0	$ (1,500)
	Year 1	$ 310
	Year 2	$ 400
	Year 3	$ 500
	Year 4	$ 750
net present value	NPV	$78.16

FIGURE J.14 Calculating NPV with an initial investment in Year 0.

Internal Rate of Return (IRR)

Internal rate of return (IRR) is the rate of growth a project is expected to generate and discount rate at which the present value of the costs of a project is equal to the present value of its expected revenue or the rate that produces a net present value of zero. Entering "IRR" into the formula window and this time selecting all of the cash flows from Year 0 through Year 4 results in a 10% IRR or the rate to compare with other investment opportunities as displayed in Figure J.15.

C10 | fx =IRR(C4:C8)

Excel	Formula	Data
rate	I	?
cash flows	CF	
	Year 0	$ (1,500)
	Year 1	$ 310
	Year 2	$ 400
	Year 3	$ 500
	Year 4	$ 750
internal rate of return	IRR	10%

FIGURE J.15 Calculating internal rate of return (IRR).

Given that the 8% interest rate from the NPV example in Figure J.14 is less than the required 10% IRR, the project should be rejected based on financial performance.

References

1. Formulas and functions. Excel Easy. http://www.excel-easy.com/introduction/formulas
   -functions.html
2. Excelfunctions.Lynda.com(LinkedIn).http://www.lynda.com/search?q=excel+functions

Index

Printed in the United States
by Baker & Taylor Publisher Services